the
Great
Cholesterol
Con

the
Great
Cholesterol
Con

**THE TRUTH ABOUT WHAT REALLY CAUSES HEART
DISEASE AND HOW TO AVOID IT**

DR MALCOLM KENDRICK

JB

First published in the UK by John Blake Publishing
an imprint of Bonnier Books UK
The Plaza,
535 Kings Road,
London SW10 0SZ
Owned by Bonnier Books
Sveavägen 56, Stockholm, Sweden

www.facebook.com/johnblakebooks
twitter.com/jblakebooks

First published in paperback in 2007

Paperback ISBN: 978-1-84454-610-7
Ebook ISBN: 978-1-84358-236-6

British Library Cataloguing-in-Publication Data:

A catalogue record for this book is available from the British Library.

Design by www.envydesign.co.uk

Printed and bound in Great Britain by Clays Ltd, Elcograf S.p.A.

13 15 17 19 20 18 16 14

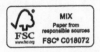

MIX
Paper from
responsible sources
FSC® C018072

John Blake Publishing is an imprint of Bonnier Books UK
www.bonnierbooks.co.uk

CONTENTS

INTRODUCTION

All humans must die... astatinate, astatinate![1]
A Dalek

We are bombarded with so much confusing nonsense about heart disease that it is difficult to know where to start. Each day that dawns, it seems, heralds a new study that flatly contradicts the last. Omega 3 fish oils are good for you; Omega 3 fish oils are not good for you. Alcohol protects against heart disease; alcohol does not protect against heart disease. Coffee is good for you; coffee is bad for you. Or maybe it was excess milk in the diet, or green-leaf tea, or... To quote my lovely daughter, 'yeah, whatever'.

It has reached the point where I feel like shouting, 'Listen guys, I know you need to 'publish or perish', and the more publicity you can achieve the bigger the next research budget, but you're scaring people half to death. No one knows what to do or what to believe any more. And by the way, your study was RUBBISH! Now go away, grow your beard, and do some proper boring research that no one can understand.'

But they won't. For it's so much more fun to appear on a news programme, talking earnestly about your discovery of the latest possible cause of heart attacks – a danger that the public absolutely, positively, must be warned about. Afterwards, you will probably be invited to lucrative speaking engagements at international cardiology

---

1 Adapted from *Dr Who and the Daleks* (1965). Screenplay by Milton Subotsky. Based on the BBC Television serial by Terry Nation. Produced by Milton Subotsky and Max J Rosenberg.

conferences. Does a professorship beckon? 'Who, me? I really don't deserve it, but if you must...'

Somehow, in this ever-changing, ever-confusing world, one idea has stood the test of time. And it is this:

The Diet-Heart Hypothesis
(aka The Cholesterol Hypothesis)

If you eat too much food containing cholesterol and/or saturated fat, the level of cholesterol in your blood will rise. The excess cholesterol will be deposited in artery walls, causing them to thicken and narrow. In time this will block blood supply to the heart (and other organs) causing a heart attack, or stroke.

Whichever name you use for it, this hypothesis has the advantage of being extra-super straightforward – suitable for children from the age of five upwards, no parental guidance required. But be careful. Perhaps the single greatest prejudice in scientific research – the researcher's holy grail, if you like – is the belief that, in the end, the simplest solutions are correct. Occam's razor, $E=MC^2$, the perfect four base sequence of DNA. But it is as well to remember a warning from history:

> *For every complicated problem there is a solution that is simple, direct, understandable and wrong.*
>
> HL Mencken

And boy, is the cholesterol hypothesis wrong. To adapt a quote from Blackadder, 'It is wronger than a very wrong thing.' Yet it has mesmerised scientists, doctors and the general public for years, exuding a siren song that none can resist, dragging us all to our doom on the sharp rocks of illogicality.

OK, when you look at the eye-watering profits being generated, it hasn't exactly dragged pharmaceutical companies to their doom – yet.

Indeed, once everyone believed that a high cholesterol level was the most important single cause of heart disease, the gold rush was on to discover drugs that could lower cholesterol levels. A highly successful gold rush led by big pharmaceutical companies.

Admittedly, at first things didn't go too well. Various substances were discovered in the 1960s and 1970s that, to widespread rejoicing, lowered cholesterol levels. However, when the clinical trials were carried out it was found that more people died when they took the drugs than when they took the placebo. In some cases the cholesterol-lowering agents very nearly doubled the overall mortality rate. Which did put rather a dampener on proceedings.

In 1970, a study by the WHO (the World Health Organization, not the rock group) on clofibrate (a big drug at the time, but now defunct for reasons that will shortly become apparent), measured blood cholesterol in 30,000 healthy, middle-aged men in Edinburgh, Prague and Budapest. The 10,000 men with the highest blood cholesterol levels were selected for the trial – half to receive clofibrate, half placebo. After five years there had been a total of 128 deaths in the clofibrate group and 87 in the placebo group. Oops. And there were more fatal heart attacks in the clofibrate group too.

It was decreed, however, that this problem had nothing whatsoever to do with the cholesterol-lowering ability of clofibrate. Perish the very thought. The drug obviously had some other, nasty, heart-disease-causing effects – not that anyone was quite sure what these effects were. But because everyone already 'knew' that a high cholesterol level caused heart disease, no one dared suggest that these results might – just might – contradict the cholesterol hypothesis. Hey ho, let not the facts spoil a good story.

The 1960s, 1970s and 1980s represented a period that could be known as the BS era; the time Before Statins began. (In a nutshell, statins are drugs that lower cholesterol and so, in the eyes of the mainstream medical community, are believed to reduce the risk of heart disease. More on this subject – much more – to follow.)

In this period new drugs were found; they lowered cholesterol, but increased mortality and were, frankly, worse than useless. I think it is true to say that the faith of the cholesterol brotherhood was becoming sorely tested. Even the pharmaceutical industry was, with extreme reluctance, heading off in different directions. Just to give one example: I find it amusing to keep a copy of a document produced by pharmaceutical giants Pfizer in 1992. This was a couple of years before 'statinomania' achieved lift-off. The document was called 'Pathologic Triggers: New Insights Into Cardiovascular Risk'. I may have the only remaining copy of this document. As such it must be worth... ooh, 50p at least.

The document begins:

> Today, most of our attempts to prevent atherosclerosis [disease of the arteries] have centered on the control of hypertension and hyperlipidaemia [raised blood pressure and raised cholesterol, respectively], as well as lifestyle factors. However, recent insights into the pathology of coronary disease have sharpened our focus on the natural history of atheroma [build-up of fatty deposits on the lining of arteries] and its relentless progression to acute cardiac events...

Curiouser and curiouser. What could they mean? In fact, throughout this document Pfizer is carefully preparing the ground for an entirely new concept: that it is not really high blood pressure and high cholesterol levels that cause heart disease – it is something else. But what could this something else be?

What indeed. According to 'New Insights into Cardiovascular Risk', heart disease is mainly associated with the formation of abnormal blood clots...

> Given the insidious nature of atherosclerosis, it is vital to consider the role of platelets [small blood cells involved in blood clotting] and thrombosis [the formation of blood clots within a blood vessel or the heart] in the process...

Today, together with the rest of the industry, they would dismiss such talk of platelets and thrombosis as utter bunk – for today we have statins. If anyone mentioned platelets now they would be told to pick up their pay cheque on the way past reception.

And how were statins discovered – these glorious and magical pills that will turn us all into latter-day Methuselahs, living well into our sixth centuries? Were they discovered by highly trained scientists toiling in research laboratories, deep in the bowels of a major pharmaceutical company? Were they discovered using three-dimensional modelling and a detailed understanding of the inner workings of liver biochemistry? Do they, indeed, represent another glorious vindication of the value of the industry's much-vaunted multi-billion-dollar research and development budget? Ah… no. As with many of the best-selling drugs, statins were discovered completely by accident.

Which takes us to a small valley in northern China. It is a cold place, a lonely place, a place where a small plant clings to existence in a hostile world (all right, I'm using a bit of poetic license here…) a plant known as red yeast rice. Red yeast rice has to deal with the many predators who find it rather tasty, making its tenuous hold on life even more precarious. But this plucky little plant has a trick up its sleeve. It produces a poison, known as lovastatin, which kills those animals that are foolish enough to eat it. A researcher from the US government discovered this plant, with its poison, and took it away for further study[2,3].

Presumably, lovastatin was a pretty useless poison, at least from the US Army's point of view. Interestingly, however, lovastatin was found to block an enzyme known as HMG-CoA reductase. This enzyme takes effect on the long, long pathway of cholesterol synthesis in the liver. Therefore, in lesser, not terribly poisonous doses, lovastatin blocks cholesterol production, and lowers blood cholesterol levels in human beings.

2 Yg, Li. Zhang, F. Wang, ZT. Hu, ZB. 'Identification and chemical profiling of monacolins in red yeast rice using high-performance liquid chromatography with photodiode array detection and mass spectrometry'. J Pharm Biomed Anal, 3 September 2004; 35(5); 1101–12.
3 Thompson, Richard. 'Foundations for blockbuster drugs in federally sponsored research', The FASEB Journal, 2001; 15; 1671–76.

Merck – for many years the world's biggest pharmaceutical company – managed to obtain lovastatin from the US Army, file a patent, and the rest – as they say – is history. Mankind had entered 'The age of the statin'. Cue celestial music – *Star Wars* theme music meets Beethoven's 'Ode to Joy', that sort of thing.

And lo it was written that Merck, clutching the great staff of Mevacor (the brand name of lovastatin) led the chosen opinion leaders to the Holy Land, a land of great bounty, where fruit hung low from the trees. A land of milk and honey where – if you were a cardiologist lucky enough to run a clinical trial on statins – huge extensions and swimming pools miraculously appeared next to your house.

And the year of 'statination' was 1987, in which Merck launched lovastatin. And there was a great wailing and gnashing of teeth from other pharmaceutical companies, who had missed a trick. But they rapidly whipped their research bods into action, crying, 'Find me another HMG-CoA enzyme inhibitor, or else you shall be cast into the outer darkness.'

Thus, over the years, several other 'statins' have appeared. Merck tripped over another one called simvastatin (now sold over the counter as Zocor Heart Pro, in the UK). Bristol-Myers Squibb (BMS) stumbled across pravastatin. Fluvastatin landed at the feet of Ciba (now part of Novartis). Warner Lambert found atorvastatin lying in a small basket in the rushes, then sold marketing rights to Pfizer. Worst business decision ever made? Atorvastatin is the world's biggest-selling drug, with profits that would make your eyes water.

Bayer mixed the wrong chemicals together and discovered cerivastatin* – so powerful that it allegedly killed hundreds of patients and had to be withdrawn (multi-billion-dollar lawsuits pending). Most recently, we have had rosuvastatin (Crestor), synthesized in Japan, sold to AstraZeneca, and marketed with ruthless determination.

All of these drugs make billions and billions of dollars of profit for their companies.

---

* Yes, I know, it was probably all a bit more scientific than this. Or maybe not. After all, GlaxoSmithKline desperately tried to develop a statin for years, and failed, despite their multi-gazillion-dollar research facilities.

At first, doctors weren't that keen on statins. Many of them didn't believe in the cholesterol hypothesis, and were far from certain that lowering cholesterol levels would do much good. However, the statin companies embarked on a series of massive clinical studies to 'prove' that lowering cholesterol with statins would work. These studies all went under a series of painfully constructed acronyms. For example:

- 4S: the Scandinavian Simvastatin Survival Study. Carried out on 4,444 patients. (Was this a contrived number or what? I am interested to know what happened to patient number 4,445? Did the door slam shut in his face? Was he left – horror of horrors – unstatinated?)
- WOSCOPS: the West Of Scotland COronary Prevention Study, which was the other really big study of the time.

The way things are going in medical research, first you have to think up a catchy acronym. Only then you can work out what study you're going to do. All very Hollywood and PR driven. Someone told me that a recent film, *It's All Gone Pete Tong*, started with the title, the location and then the budget, before anyone had written a screenplay. Then there's the *Haunted Mansion*, a film based on a ride in Disneyworld Florida. How about *Chewing Gum*, a film based on a bit of muck I just found on the bottom on my shoe?

Anyway, 4S and WOSCOPS were two of the earliest, and most influential statin studies (4S came out in 1994, WOSCOPS the following year). Since then we have had many others: TEXCAPS, AFCAPS, J-LIT, CARE, ASCOT, PROSPER, ALLHAT, A to Z, PROVE-IT, TNT et cetera, et cetera. The mind boggles and it becomes very difficult to remember which results came from which study.

Whatever the acronym, all of these studies have been presented as a glorious vindication of the cholesterol hypothesis and of the value of statins. Here are just two comments from experts following the publication of the 4S and WOSCOPS studies. They pretty much sum up mainstream thinking in the area.

My takeaway for clinicians is that we now have two very well designed, very well run, large randomized clinical trials in the last two years that provide us with rock solid evidence that in patients with elevated cholesterol that have either CHD [coronary heart disease] or multiple risk factors that lowering cholesterol aggressively with statins reduces cardiac mortality, cardiac morbidity and it reduces overall mortality. And therefore, the controversy which is surrounding this area, with these clear results, should really be put to rest.

J Sanford Schwartz, MD, Executive Director
of the Leonard Davis Institute of Health
Economics at the University of Pennsylvania

The greater the cholesterol lowering the greater the reduction in clinical events. This has been shown by taking all the trials and putting the results together. The more recent trials with the statin drugs, we can lower cholesterol much better than with older drugs, and get much better results.

Scott Grundy, MD, director and chairman,
Centre for Human Nutrition, The University of
Texas Southwestern Medical Center at Dallas

You get the general drift.

So, finally, a class of drugs had been found that lowered cholesterol levels, protected against heart disease, and didn't kill people at the same time – hallelujah! 'On this basis, I put it to the members of the jury that the cholesterol hypothesis had been proven, beyond doubt. This court must convict cholesterol of crimes against humanity, m'lord.'

Judge (placing black cap on his head): 'I order that this sad and dangerous chemical be taken from this place, to another place, where it shall be hanged by the neck, until dead. May God have mercy on its soul.'

At this point, I feel a bit like Henry Fonda in *Twelve Angry Men*. We seem to have travelled far beyond the realm of the scientific hypothesis, to the land of 'known fact': it now seems beyond argument that raised cholesterol levels cause heart disease, and that statins are wonderful, life-enhancing drugs.

Yet I think we have been sold a pup. A rather large pup – more of a full-grown blue whale, in fact. But how can I convince you, my fellow jurors, of the truth? You have heard so much, read so much, listened to experts promoting the wonders of statins and ever-greater cholesterol lowering. Adverts bombard us every day with some new fabulous yoghurt, probiotic, margarine or milk drink assuring us that these things lower cholesterol, thus protecting your heart.

On the basis of this never-ending information, many of you will be convinced that you should take statins for the rest of your natural lifespan. Firstly, of course, you will be frightened into action by a blood test demonstrating that you – you sinner – have a raised cholesterol level ('Have you been eating hamburgers again? Have you?'). Everywhere you look, everybody is in agreement about the need to lower your cholesterol level. How can almost everybody be wrong?

In fact, almost everybody being wrong has been a quite normal phenomenon throughout human existence. So the fact that there are only a few dissenting voices out there shouldn't bother you unduly. And medical scientists (an oxymoron if ever there was one), have a long and distinguished history of grabbing entirely the wrong end of the stick, closing their eyes tightly shut, holding on grimly and refusing to listen to anybody else. Another leech anybody, or perhaps a radical mastectomy, or a tonsillectomy, or a removal of toxic colon? What about that old chestnut 'no bacteria can live in the human stomach'? And 'strict bed rest following a heart attack' – how many millions did that kill?

The list of stupid, damaging and plain wrong things that doctors have been taught over the years makes rather depressing reading. It has certainly depressed me from time to time. We can all be wrong. Even me. But for some reason, the medical hierarchy is exceptionally reluctant to admit their mistakes. I think it's a control-freak thing. You know, transactional analysis: doctor/stern parent, patient/naughty child. Me… three-year-old having a tantrum.

Anyway, back to the discussion. Here are the facts that I hope to convince you are true:

> **1: A high-fat diet, saturated or otherwise, has no impact on blood cholesterol levels.**
>
> **2: Fact one is unimportant, because…**
>
> **3: High cholesterol levels don't cause heart disease anyway (the second part of the cholesterol hypothesis is wrong).**
>
> **4: Statins do not protect against heart disease by lowering cholesterol levels – they work in another way.**
>
> **5: The protection provided by statins is so small as to be not worth bothering about for most people (and all women). The reality is that the benefits have been hyped beyond belief.**
>
> **6: Statins have many more unpleasant side effects than has been admitted. Side-effects up to, and including, death and the creation of horribly deformed babies. (You think not? Then read on.)**
>
> **7: 'Experts' in this area should not be listened to, because they are all paid ridiculous sums of money by statin manufacturers to sing loudly from a prepared hymn sheet. Every single one of them – apart from me, obviously.**

I hope that once you have read this book, the vast majority of you will cast off your statins and walk again. For those not taking statins: you can tell your doctor to stick them where the sun doesn't shine. (And no, they do not make a suppository version.) This could save the NHS at least £2 billion a year, and prevent hundreds of thousand of people from suffering unpleasant side effects, and being turned into lifelong hypochondriacs.

Not only this, but I shall then tell you what really does cause heart disease. So you get two books for the price of one. Unfortunately, for those of you who like such things, the answer is not a 'five minutes a day to prevent heart disease' solution. Nor a 'West Coast' diet, nor a 'Hip and Thigh' diet. It is rather more complicated than that. Sorry.

You may not think it now. But by the time you have read this book, you will be convinced that I am right, and everyone else is wrong. I say this with all necessary humility.

I am not alone in my beliefs. There are many hundreds of doctors and researchers who agree that the cholesterol hypothesis is bunk. Many keep their counsel, others have been stomped into silence, but a few have had the guts to speak out. However, their voices, unlike those of the implacable medical 'statinators', are not supported by multi-billion-dollar pharmaceutical budgets.

In a world dominated by PR-controlled spin, critics of the cholesterol hypothesis get very little airtime. If they did, this world would change, and I hope this book starts the process of change. Because, despite my apparent joviality, I am deadly serious in my belief that the misguided war against cholesterol, using statins, represents something very close to a crime against humanity. So close that you may not be able to spot the difference.

CHAPTER 1

WHAT IS HEART DISEASE, ANYWAY?

The main underlying theme of this book is heart disease – what causes it and what doesn't. But the term 'heart disease' is virtually meaningless. A pedant would say that heart disease is a 'disease of the heart', but there are hundreds of them, most with complex names – myocarditis, pericarditis, ventricular hypertrophy, Woff-Parkinson-White Syndrome, to name but four.

However, the big daddy, the one that kills most people, is not truly a

Fig. 1 Blockage in right coronal artery

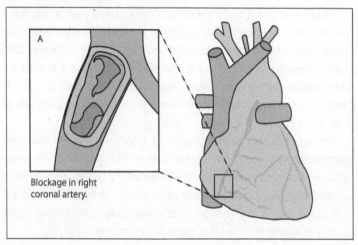

A

Blockage in right
coronal artery.

disease of the heart at all. It is a disease of the arteries that supply blood to the heart, and is usually called atherosclerosis. 'Athero', or 'atheroma', describes the build up of grey-white/fatty gunk in the artery walls. These thickenings are sometimes called atheromatous plaques, or just plaques. 'Sclerosis' means general thickening and hardening. One of the other confusing elements when reading about heart disease is the amount of jargon. AKA medical terminology.

Atheromatous plaques come in many different varieties. The American Heart Association even has a grading system from one to five, and then further subsections into type 5(i) and 5(ii)... and probably type 4(B), subsection (ii) paragraph 6. You get the picture.

Plaques are generally thought to progress from an initial 'fatty streak', as found in the arteries of most ten-year-olds, which gradually becomes bigger and thicker. Eventually, the plaques can reach the point where they actually calcify, turning arteries into stiff, almost bonelike tubes. The process of turning from a fatty streak into a calcified plaque is supposed to take years and years, although no one knows for sure how long things take because no one has ever hung around to watch an individual plaque going through its lifecycle (not in a human being, at least). The general assumption seems to be that it all takes decades.

Having said this, it is not the mature, stiff, calcified plaque that is the problem; it is an intermediate stage, the so-called 'unstable' plaque. At some point during their (allegedly) slow development, plaques turn into something that looks like a cyst lurking within the artery wall; a thin capsule surrounding a semi-liquid centre full of goo. This goo is made of all sorts of stuff. Fats, dead white cells, broken down bits of blood clot etc.

The great danger with this type of plaque is that the thin wall surrounding the goo bursts, or breaks down. This 'goo exposure' sends a hugely powerful message to the blood-clotting system, and results in a blood clot (also called a thrombus) forming over the burst plaque. If the blood clot is big enough then it completely blocks the blood supply to whatever organ that particular artery was supplying:

Fig. 2 Development of a blood clot in an artery

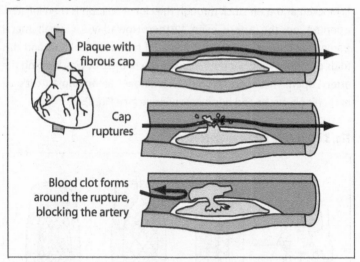

If that organ happens to be the heart, then the heart muscle downstream will become starved of oxygen. It may then 'infarct' ('infarction' means the localised necrosis – or cell death – that results from obstruction to the blood supply). In medical speak, this is a myocardial (heart muscle) infarction, often shortened to an MI. In layperson speak, this is a heart attack. It is estimated that about 50 per cent of heart attacks are fatal, and people mostly die in the first hour. For those who survive the first hour, though, a myriad of medical interventions have now been developed.

Among the earlier developments were clot-busting drugs, designed to break down the clot that is blocking the artery. These are still widely used, and are pretty effective – assuming you managed to 'bust' the clot before the heart muscle became too badly damaged. That said, the humble blood-thinning aspirin can be almost as good, at about one-millionth of the cost.

However, cardiologists now have much better toys to play with, and the latest type of treatment for an acute heart attack employs a long, thin catheter, which is inserted into an artery in the groin. Under X-ray guidance; this is then fed up to the heart, directed into the artery that is blocked and then stuck through the clot. A balloon is then inflated, opening up the artery even further. Nowadays, a small metal framework known as a stent is wrapped round the balloon, and this folds out into a rigid 'support' that sits where the clot was, keeping the artery open. The entire procedure is known as angioplasty. It's all exceedingly clever, and horribly expensive (See Fig. 3).

Fig. 3 Procedure for an angioplasty

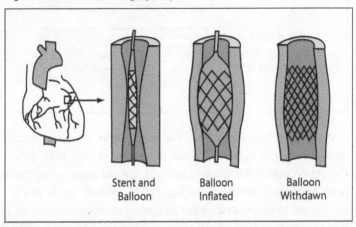

| Stent and Balloon | Balloon Inflated | Balloon Withdawn |

For those in whom clot-busters and stents haven't worked, there is the Coronary Artery Bypass Graft (CABG), or 'cabbage' – although doing a cabbage in an acute situation is pretty much the last resort of last resorts. Or, as we used to say in Scotland, TOTS, which stands for Tatties Over The Side (a tatty is a potato) – a reference to the point in a storm when the crew has to ditch the very last bit of cargo to save the ship.

Ergo, a CABG in an acute MI – when clot-busters or angioplasty hasn't worked – is TOTS time. You see, the jargon is quite simple once you get the hang of it.

Quite how much impact all of this cleverness has had on overall mortality rates from having a heart attack is a moot point. Around fifty per cent of people die before reaching hospital, so they can't be saved.

Another forty per cent, or so, were always going to survive no matter how badly the hospital cocked up. So, at very best, these techniques can improve survival after a heart attack by about ten per cent, and we are nowhere near achieving this yet. Perhaps two or three per cent more people survive a heart attack now than about ten or twenty years ago.

Don't get me wrong. If I had a heart attack I would want a cardiologist warming up the cath lab, ready to stick a stent right up the old femoral artery. No question about it. Nothing but the best for me, thank you very much. But when it comes to heart attacks, cure is always going to be very much less impressive than prevention. Even if it is much less sexy.

Before we move on, I need to provide a little more information about 'infarctions' elsewhere in the body. Because although plaques most often develop in the arteries supplying blood to the heart (coronary arteries), plaques are perfectly capable of developing elsewhere in the body too. Quite often, big plaques form in the arteries in the neck (carotid arteries). As these arteries supply blood to the brain, this is clearly a danger spot. However, the carotid arteries very rarely block completely. What most often happens is that a clot forms over the carotid plaque, then a bit breaks off and travels up into the brain through ever-smaller arteries.

Once the clot reaches an artery that is too narrow for it, it gets stuck, and this dams up blood supply to an area of the brain, leading to a cerebral (brain) infarction. This is the commonest version of a 'stroke'. The other type of stroke occurs when an artery in the brain bursts, causing a bleed into the brain tissue. This is called a cerebral haemorrhage.

In fact, one of the reasons why it has been so hard to develop an effective treatment for stroke is that, clinically, it is impossible to tell the difference between an infarct/blockage, and a bleed/haemorrhage. You need to do a brain scan to know, for sure, what type of stroke has occurred. You can't give a clot-busting drug to someone having a stroke, because, if they are having a 'bleed', the drugs will make things far, far, worse. In fact, you will almost certainly kill them. And, by the time you have managed to get a brain scan done, it is usually too late to give any drug at all, because the damage will already have been done.

Moving on from that cheery subject. Apart from the heart and the brain, you can have infarctions in the kidneys, the guts, the eyes – almost anywhere, in fact. (At this point, it occurs to me that I should, perhaps, have inscribed the words DON'T PANIC on the cover of the book.)

Perhaps the scariest place to develop big plaques is in the aorta, the major blood vessel that leads out of the heart and down through the chest and abdomen. If the aorta develops big plaques, the wall can lose structural integrity and balloon outwards, creating a great big 'aneurysm' (see Fig. 4). This is like having an unexploded bomb in your chest, just waiting to go off. And when an artery this big fails – kaboom! In medical speak, this is known as a ruptured aortic aneurysm. In general, it is something to be avoided. Some people survive – so long as the leak is small, that is.

Fig. 4 Comparison between normal aorta and aorta with aneurysm

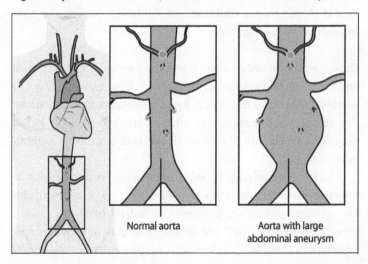

Normal aorta

Aorta with large abdominal aneurysm

SUMMARY OF FACTS

- Heart disease is really a disease of the arteries supplying blood to the heart.

- The 'disease' is atherosclerosis (or the development of discrete atherosclerotic plaques).

- Plaques can also develop in arteries almost anywhere in the body.

- Plaques are dangerous when they burst, or 'rupture', as this stimulates the formation of a blood clot over the ruptured area. This can completely block the artery, causing the tissue downstream to infarct.

POSTSCRIPT

Nothing written in this chapter is contentious. It is all broadly accepted and represents mainstream thinking and research. Although, as with everything scientific, there are bound to be points where some people would say 'That's not quite true' or 'I disagree with that description.'

However... however. I would hate to give the impression that everything is quite as simple as I have indicated. The reality is that nothing in the area of heart disease is pure black and white. Here are three facts for you to ponder.

Fact one:
A post-mortem study found that a group of Japanese had the same degree of atherosclerosis in their arteries as a group of American men. Yet the rate of death from heart disease in the Japanese example was one-sixth that of America in middle-aged men and women. At least, it was at the time of the study 'Comparison of aortic atherosclerosis

in the United States, Japan and Guatemala', by Gore I, Hirst AE and Koseki Y (American Journal of Clinical Nutrition, 1959; 7:50-54).

Fact two:
In the majority of cases, the blood clot (thrombus) thought to have triggered the heart attack will have formed days, or even weeks, before the heart attack itself. Does this mean that acute blockage of a coronary artery does not cause a heart attack? (An addendum to fact two is that, in many cases, no blockage in an artery can be found at post-mortem.)

Fact three:
Men who dig out coal in very deep mines in Russia often die very young from heart attacks. The average age at death is 41. Yes, 41. On autopsy, most of them show signs of several previous heart attacks, yet few of them have any history of having had a heart attack, or chest pains. Does this mean that most heart attacks do not cause chest pain?

Finally, to emphasise the point that things are far more complicated – and far more interesting – than the current almost mechanical view of heart disease and heart attacks (according to which the arteries are seen as a pipe carrying blood, and the heart as a simple pump), consider the following.

A myocardial infarction is defined as 'localised necrosis resulting from obstruction to the blood supply.' Sounds simple, but think again. 'Necrosis' means tissue death. Below, I have included a picture of the end result of frostbite. In frostbite, areas of the body – particularly the fingers or toes – freeze, then become blackened and dead, and finally fall off. They are often referred to as 'necrotic areas'.

Imagine, for a moment, what would happen if the bit of heart muscle affected by a lack of blood supply – the area of myocardial infarction – actually did die, as in frostbite. You would end up with a blackened, dead bit of heart muscle that would then, inevitably, fall off. At which point you would have a big hole in the side of your heart. Which, I think I can state with absolute confidence, would be 100 per cent fatal.

Fig. 5 Injuries resulting from frostbite

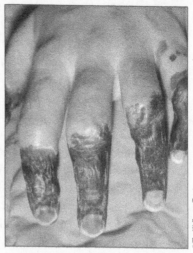

© The Wellcome Trust

But this does not happen – ever. What happens is that the area of infarcted tissue changes from muscle, which requires a lot of oxygen to function, into a form of scar tissue, which can survive on very little oxygen. In short, heart muscle does not actually become necrotic, or die, following a heart attack. Instead, what happens is a process of cell alteration, or adaptation – which means that, at some point, the cells affected by a lack of blood supply are deciding whether or not to 'infarct' and change into scar tissue or, instead, to remain as fully functioning heart muscle. How and why do they make this decision? Who knows.

What we do know, however, is that in people with established heart disease you can find regions of the heart where muscle is 'hibernating'. It hasn't converted to scar tissue, but it isn't contracting either. It's simply sitting and waiting. Waiting for what? For the blood supply to recover, presumably. How long can heart muscle wait like this? Quite a long time. Weeks at least, perhaps months, maybe years.

I hope this example makes it clear that 'heart attacks' are far from simple things whereby a pipe (the artery) blocks up, oxygen supply dries up and muscle then dies. It is true that the artery blocks up, but after that a hugely complex process swings into action that may, or may not, result in heart muscle converting into scar tissue.

In addition, the artery itself is fully capable of opening up again – which is why, presumably, the heart muscle sits 'hibernating', waiting for blood supply to return. Failing this, the heart may grow new arteries to bypass the blockage. This is known as developing 'collateral' circulation.

And the same degree of complexity goes for almost every other aspect of heart disease. Thus, atherosclerosis is not a case of a pipe gradually thickening with cholesterol, like a central-heating system clogging up. This seems a nice simple analogy, but it is hopelessly flawed. Take, for example, this cutting from the Savannah *Morning News*. Don't ask me anything about this newspaper – I was sent the cutting by a fellow cholesterol sceptic, as it seemed to him the perfect example of a stupid analogy:

> *Photos taken inside clogged city sewer pipes look nearly identical to medical photos of the blood vessels of patients who have spent a lifetime gorging on fried chicken, sausage, and bacon. 'It's like your arteries,' said John Parker, environmental compliance inspector with the city's Water and Sewer Department. 'Grease builds up in there. It's gory.' And just like in the body, clogs can form little by little, the accumulation of lots of neighbors each sending a little grease down the drain.*

There are so many ways in which this analogy is wrong, that I just can't possibly outline them all here. Hopefully, by the time you have finished this book you will understand that anyone making such a statement needs to be taken out and slapped repeatedly with a wet kipper.

CHAPTER 2

WHAT IS CHOLESTEROL, ANYWAY?
(And what's a fat?)

Cholesterol has been a favourite theme on the airwaves for the past 30 years, and mostly it seems to get a pretty harsh press. Here is what BUPA have to say about cholesterol on their website.

> The main risk associated with high cholesterol is coronary heart disease [CHD]. This is caused by blood vessels becoming narrowed with fatty deposits called plaques, which cholesterol contributes to. The narrowed blood vessels reduce blood flow to the heart. This can result in angina [chest pain] or, if the vessel is blocked completely, a heart attack. For more information see the BUPA factsheets on Angina and Heart Attack.

Based on information such as this, most people naturally think of cholesterol as something damaging, something to be avoided. But I think it is important to make it clear that cholesterol is absolutely essential for life. It is not some alien chemical that we can remove from our diets, or our bodies.

On this topic, I was amused to read an article in the *Independent* newspaper about the Buncefield Depot fire (when much of Britain's fuel stores went up in smoke, if you remember). This article highlighted the dangers in the fire-fighting foam that was used, which contains perfluorooctane sulfonate (PFOS). Among the serial terrors of PFOS was the fact that… 'The chemical is believed to interrupt the body's ability to produce cholesterol, a necessary building block of nearly every system in the body.' Quite.

I sometimes remark to those who think my ideas on heart disease are entirely batty, 'Why do you think that an egg yolk is full of cholesterol?' Answer: because it takes one hell of a lot of cholesterol to build a healthy chicken. It also takes a hell of a lot of cholesterol to build, and maintain, a healthy human being. In fact, cholesterol is so vital that all cells, apart from neurones, can manufacture cholesterol, and one of the key functions of the liver is to synthesize cholesterol. We also have an entire transportation system dedicated to moving cholesterol around the body.

Effects of Smith-Lemli-Opitz Syndrome (SLOS)

Spontaneous abortion of fetuses with SLOS is not unusual. Stillbirths have also been reported.

Death from multi-organ system failure during the first weeks of life is typical in individuals with SLOS type II.

Congenital heart disease is not uncommon in SLOS and can cause cyanosis and congestive heart failure.

Vomiting, feeding difficulties, constipation, toxic megacolon, electrolyte disturbances and failure to thrive are common and, in some cases, related to gastrointestinal anomalies.

Visual loss may occur because of cataracts, optic-nerve abnormalities, or other ophthalmologic problems.

Hearing loss is fairly common.

Cause of death can include pneumonia, lethal congenital heart defect, or hepatic failure. Survival is unlikely if the plasma cholesterol level is less than approximately 20mg/dL.

To highlight what happens when cholesterol levels are very low, it is enlightening to look at a rare genetic condition called Smith-Lemli-Opitz Syndrome (SLOS). In this syndrome there is a defect in cholesterol synthesis, resulting in very low blood cholesterol levels. Listed opposite are some of the effects. For more information visit http://www.emedecine.com/ped/topic2117.htm

From this cheery little list of deadly abnormalities, at least one thing becomes clear. The only good cholesterol molecule is *not* a dead cholesterol molecule. A very, very low cholesterol level is not something we should strive too hard to achieve.

Moving on, here are some of the things that we need cholesterol for in the body:

- Brain synapses. Synapses, the vital connections between nerve cells in the brain, and elsewhere, are made almost entirely of cholesterol.

- Vitamin D. This is a highly important vitamin, not only needed to create healthy bones, but now also known to be protective against a number of cancers. Vitamin D is synthesized from cholesterol by the action of sunlight on our skin.

- Cell membranes. All cells in our body need cholesterol in their cell membranes. Without it they would disintegrate, as cholesterol provides structural integrity.

- Sex hormones. Cholesterol is a building block for most sex hormones.

- Bile. Cholesterol is a key component of bile, which is released from the gall bladder to help with food digestion. Indeed, many gallstones are made entirely from crystallised cholesterol.

It should be pointed out that all of this requires a great deal cholesterol. So much so that it is nigh on impossible to eat enough cholesterol to meet your daily cholesterol needs. In order to meet this gap, the liver has to produce four or five times as much cholesterol as you ingest. In fact, you would need to eat about six to eight egg yolks each and every day to meet your daily requirement. As most of us never do this, the liver fills the gap.

So how can it possibly make sense to claim that eating, say, one-third of our daily cholesterol requirement (which would only happen if you nearly doubled your intake) - instead of the normal one-fifth, or one-sixth, that most people manage - will overwhelm our metabolic control systems, causing cholesterol levels to spiral out of control? If we did managed to eat four eggs a day, the liver would simply produce less cholesterol to keep the levels steady.

This form of physiological 'downregulation', also known as a 'negative feedback system', is something found in all other biological systems, in all other organisms discovered to date. But not, it would appear, with cholesterol, according to the 'cholesterol is bad' theory.

However much cholesterol you eat, the liver just keeps churning away, manufacturing as much as ever. Hmmmm, let me think. This would be like... Actually it would be just like nothing else at all ever discovered in nature, ever. (I'll return to this subject later.)

* * * * *

Now it is time to move on to fats, with a special focus on our friendly neighbourhood saturated fat - aka the mass murderer. Saturated fats, so we are repeatedly informed, raise our cholesterol levels, thus killing us all from heart disease. 'Super-size me, baby, one more time...' In addition to this, they have also been implicated in causing cancer and diabetes, and other nasty conditions too numerous to mention.

So I think it is time to reveal this monster of the deep.

Fig. 6 Saturated fat

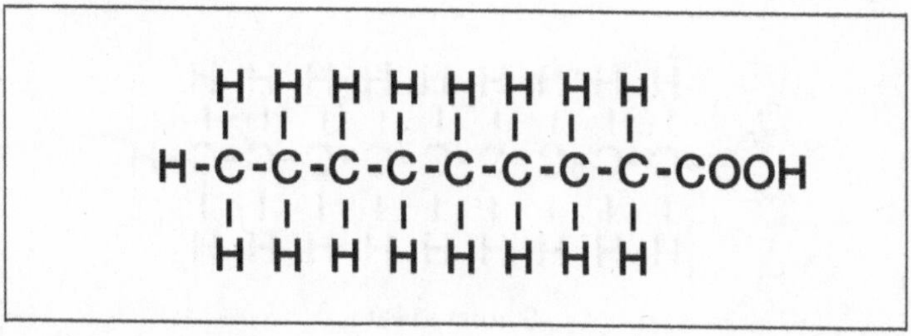

$$
\begin{array}{c}
\text{H}\ \ \text{H}\ \ \text{H}\ \ \text{H}\ \ \text{H}\ \ \text{H}\ \ \text{H}\ \ \text{H} \\
|\ \ \ \ |\ \ \ \ |\ \ \ \ |\ \ \ \ |\ \ \ \ |\ \ \ \ |\ \ \ \ | \\
\text{H}-\text{C}-\text{C}-\text{C}-\text{C}-\text{C}-\text{C}-\text{C}-\text{C}-\text{COOH} \\
|\ \ \ \ |\ \ \ \ |\ \ \ \ |\ \ \ \ |\ \ \ \ |\ \ \ \ |\ \ \ \ | \\
\text{H}\ \ \text{H}\ \ \text{H}\ \ \text{H}\ \ \text{H}\ \ \text{H}\ \ \text{H}\ \ \text{H}
\end{array}
$$

Eeeeeeeehhhhhh! Run for the hills, hide your children, cover your eyes! Here, in all its terrifying glory, is a saturated fat. The greatest killer in the western world.

OK, I know what you're thinking. Is that it? Yup, that's it. Saturated fats are among the simplest of all molecules in the body. They contain carbon, oxygen and hydrogen, and they all have a COOH group at one end. They can be rather longer than the one in the diagram – i.e. they can have a longer chain of carbon atoms, each with two hydrogen atoms attached. Or they can be shorter. But that's about as exciting as saturated fats get.

So what is it about this substance that is so deadly? Frankly, I'm the wrong person to ask, because I don't happen to think that saturated fats are in any way damaging or dangerous. If they were, they wouldn't taste so damn delicious. Nature tends to warn us off dangerous foods by making them taste bitter and icky. Or giving them a bright-red colour. But hey, I know the counter argument in all its Darwinian glory: nature doesn't care about us after we are too old to procreate, so things that kill us after the age of 50 don't matter. I refuse to enter this debate because it is neither winnable, nor loseable. You either accept it, or reject it, according to your pre-existing philosophical prejudices.

Anyway, now you know what a saturated fat is, perhaps I should introduce you to an unsaturated fat, those tree-hugging, Gaia-loving, spiritual healers of all mankind – sorry, humankind.

Fig. 7 Comparison of a saturated fat and an unsaturated fat

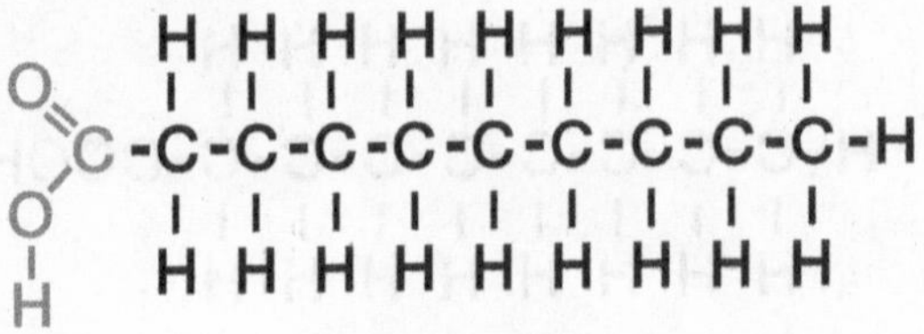

Saturated Fat

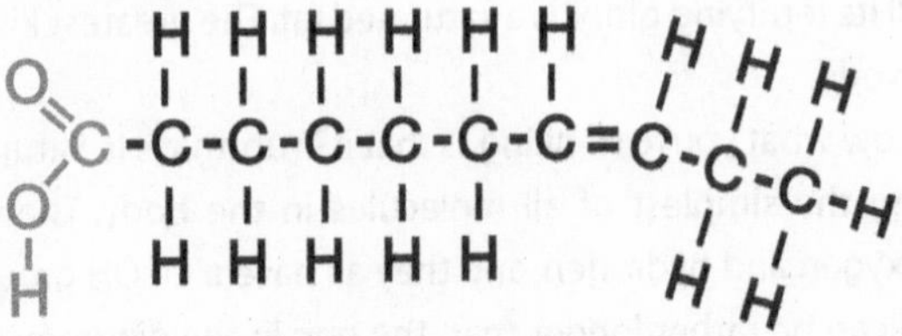

Unsaturated Fat

Can you spot the difference between a saturated and unsaturated fat? The difference is that a section of the unsaturated fat is missing two hydrogen atoms. With two hydrogen atoms missing, a double bond has formed between two carbon atoms in the chain. Because this fat has a double bond in the middle of it, it is deemed to be not fully 'saturated' with hydrogen atoms. Thus, it is 'unsaturated'.

There is something else about this particular unsaturated fat that I should point out. It is an Omega 3 fatty acid. Which is officially the healthiest molecule in the world. Indeed, you are looking at the substance that cures just about every ailment of mankind. A veritable Beecham's Powder of the early 21st century.

Perhaps I should explain exactly what makes this fat an Omega 3 fatty acid. Firstly, it is called a fatty acid because it has a COOH at one end (the acid group). In fact, all fats have this. Ergo, all fats are fatty acids, and all fatty acids are fats. But fatty acid does sound so much more scientific and clever than 'fat'. Try saying 'Omega 3 fat'. It just does not have the same ring to it. How can a fat possibly be healthy? But an 'Omega 3 fatty acid'... Now you're talking!

The 'Omega 3' refers to the position of the double bond. In the diagram above, you will notice the double bond is three carbon atoms along from the right-hand end. This end of a fat is known as the Omega end. The other end is known as the Alpha end. It's a Greek language thing: from alpha to omega, or A to Z.

I think it would be useful if I explained four more things about fats. Namely:

- What, exactly, a polyunsaturated fat is.
- How to turn a liquid fat into a solid fat (e.g. a 'cholesterol-reducing' spread).
- How fats are transported and stored in the body.
- The lack of connection between fats and cholesterol.

What is a polyunsaturated fat?

A polyunsaturated fat is a fat with more than one double bond in it. Such fats tend to come from vegetable sources, e.g. olive oil. At this point I should probably mention that a 'monounsaturated fat' is an unsaturated fat with only one double bond.

And, to be frank, that's quite enough about unsaturated fats.

How to turn a liquid fat into a solid fat

A significant problem with liquid fats (oils) is that it is kind of difficult to spread them on bread. Speaking as a butter fan, this is not something that has ever bothered me. However, many years ago, a clever chemist worked out that if you fired hydrogen atoms at great speed at an unsaturated fat, you could saturate it with a few more hydrogen atoms. The alternative chemical name for this process is hydrogenation – which literally means adding more hydrogen atoms. Whatever you call it, this chemical adaptation prevents fats from going rancid (i.e., picking up random oxygen atoms), and it also turns liquid fats into solid fats.

In this way, olive oil can be turned into olive fat – 'Zo 'ealthee as part of a Mediterranean diet.' (Cue Italian music on an accordion, with 120-year-old men dancing the tango while charming their equally ancient wives.) Just what the world always needed. Solid olive oil.

Something else that I should mention at this point is that when you fire hydrogen at unsaturated fat, you create a strange type of molecule – one that is not really found in nature at all. It is a molecule with a hydrogen atom either side of the double carbon bond. This is known as a 'trans' bond, and is a bit difficult to explain in words. So, here is a diagram:

Fig. 8 Comparison of a trans bond and a cis bond

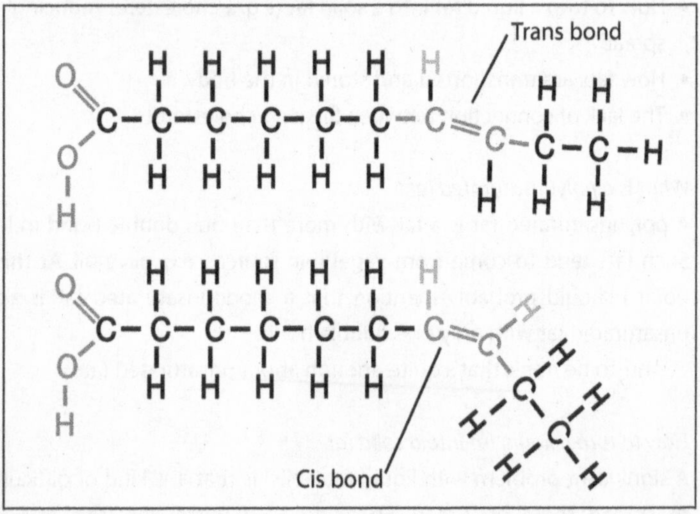

Nature tends to make all double bonds with hydrogen on the same side, which is known as a 'cis' bond. But mankind, with a big machine, extremely high pressure and a few heavy-metal catalysts, can manufacture 'trans' bonds. And fats containing trans bonds are known as 'trans-fatty acids'. There are those – and I rank myself among them – who believe that trans-fatty acids are both, literally, 'unnatural' and potentially damaging to our health.

How so? Because our enzyme systems are designed to deal with cis bonds, not trans bonds. And while the difference may seem trifling, consider the humble prion. A prion is a misfolded protein. If you eat prions from an infected source, you may develop BSE (bovine spongiform encephalopathy) and your brain will turn to mush. Ergo, unnatural differences in molecular structures can be extraordinarily damaging to biological systems – e.g. human beings.

If you want to know more about the potential damage caused by trans fats, just type 'Mary Enig' and 'trans fats' into any search engine, and be prepared to be scared. You may never eat margarine again. Despite the fact that such unnatural spreads '… are clinically proven to lower cholesterol as part of a healthy diet' – A Celebrity. ('Can I have my cheque now, please?') Ah yes, any one of the well known brands of substitute butter spreads are as natural as high-pressure, platinum-catalyst-based, hydrocarbon-cracking chemistry itself.

How fats are transported and stored around the body

I will attempt to explain fat transportation in the next chapter, as it is key to the entire batty 'high cholesterol causes heart disease hypothesis'. Here, however, I want to point out that fats do not wander through the body all alone or randomly. They are almost exclusively grouped together as three fats, attached to a backbone. Thus, they are knows as triglycerides (tri: three; glyceride: from 'glycerol' – the backbone molecule that holds the fats together).

Triglyceride

I am not entirely sure why fats do this, possibly the body finds it easier to pack three fats configured like this into smaller spaces. Also, they are less likely to react with surrounding chemicals. Whatever the main reason, this is the primary structure of fats in the body (see Fig.9.).

At this point I am going to mention a little more about glycerol, the backbone molecule in a triglyceride. Glycerol is actually half of a glucose or sugar molecule and when triglycerides are broken down into their component parts, glycerol travels to the liver, which combines two molecules to form glucose. The fats go to muscles to be burned up. (In short, stored fats are part sugar, providing energy.)

Fig. 9 Triglyceride

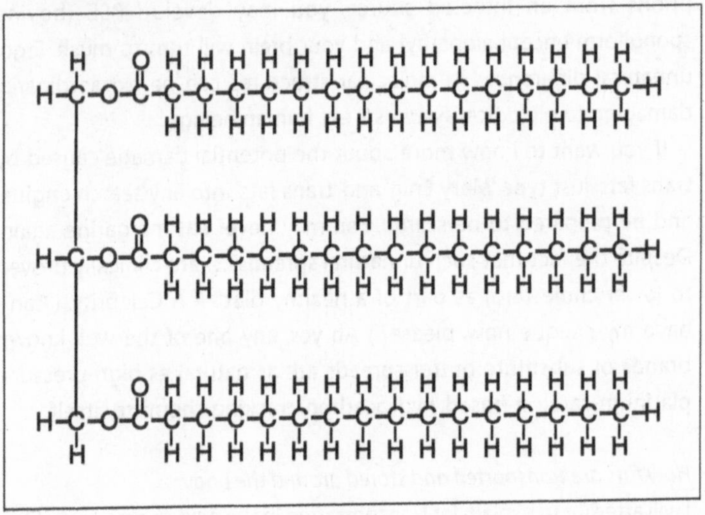

You probably do not think this matters at all. However, later on, when I attempt to explain the true cause of heart disease, this information will become rather more important.

The lack of connection between fats and cholesterol

At this point, you may have noticed that I have talked about fats and cholesterol without there seeming to be the slightest connection between them. The reason for this is because there is no connection between them. Yet the way they are discussed today, the impression seems to be given that the two things are virtually the same. Fats, cholesterol; cholesterol, fats. Low-fat diet lowers cholesterol; high-fat diet raises cholesterol… rhubarb, rhubarb.

It is true that foods containing cholesterol also tend to contain fats – specifically, saturated fat. That's because foods containing cholesterol usually come from animal sources, and so do foods containing saturated fat. This is both the beginning and the end of any dietary connection. Yet for some reason it has become a canon of medical faith that eating saturated fat raises cholesterol levels, and the two substances have become almost interchangeable in discussions on heart disease.

Here, for example, is a short passage plucked off the internet from a US governmental organisation:

> *Dietary cholesterol comes from animal sources such as egg yolks, meat (especially organ meats such as liver), poultry, fish, and higher fat milk products. Many of these foods are also high in saturated fats. Choosing foods with less cholesterol and saturated fat will help lower your blood cholesterol levels.*
>
> *http://www.nal.usda.gov/fnic/dga/dga95/lowfat.html*

Within one quick paragraph, cholesterol and saturated fats have, somehow, become inextricably intertwined.

Moving ahead of myself just for a moment, I think it might be interesting to set the above quote beside one from Ancel Keys. The name probably means nothing to you, but Keys is 'le Grand Fromage' himself. The man who, almost single-handedly, set the world implacably against saturated fat. As part of his one-man crusade against saturated fat, Ancel Keys studied the impact of cholesterol consumption on cholesterol levels in humans, and the results of his research can be neatly encapsulated in the following quote:

> *There's no connection whatsoever between cholesterol in food and cholesterol in blood. And we've known that all along. Cholesterol in the diet doesn't matter at all unless you happen to be a chicken or a rabbit.*
>
> Ancel Keys, PhD, Professor Emeritus at the
> University of Minnesota, 1997

Presumably, therefore, if cholesterol in the diet does not raise cholesterol levels – which it doesn't – it must be saturated fat? But what is the connection? Does saturated fat act as a building block for cholesterol? If you pump saturated fat into the liver, does it automatically churn out cholesterol – like inserting a pig in one end of an abattoir and watching sausages come out the other end?

I would like to say that there is absolutely no way that you can turn saturated fat (or any other sort of fat) into cholesterol. But human biochemistry is so complicated and interconnected that I can't really be so bold as to make that claim. The liver is the most fantastic chemical factory in the world. It can take almost any molecule and, through a series of mind-bogglingly complicated steps, turn it into another molecule (with certain important exceptions). So you can't say, for absolute certain, that fat doesn't become cholesterol, because some bits of fat probably do become incorporated into cholesterol, after the liver has mashed it about, and cleaved it, and added a few different atoms here and there. However, let me point out the following two facts, and leave you to draw your own conclusions.

Fact one
The fundamental building block for cholesterol is a substance called Acetyl CoA. You need know only two things about this substance:

Fig. 10 Acetyl CoA

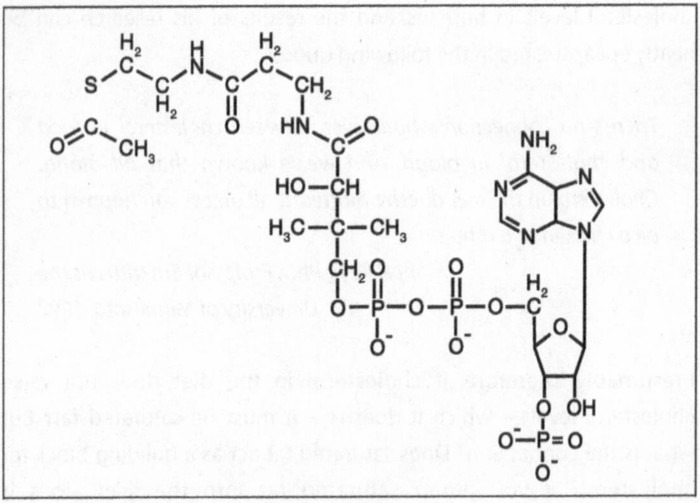

1: It contains phosphorous, sulphur and nitrogen (none of which is found in fats, they are found in proteins).

2: It has several ring structures (none of which are found in fats).

Perhaps I should start a new competition. In Fig.10 of Acetyl CoA, can you 'Spot the fat'?

Fact two

Synthesis of cholesterol is horribly complicated. Again, the purpose of Fig. 11 is simply to illustrate this fact (and also to highlight the complete absence of saturated fat anywhere in this process).

Cholesterol biosynthesis

Given these facts, I will reiterate the question: why would eating saturated fat have any impact on cholesterol production in the liver, or anywhere else in the body? If you can see how this happens, perhaps you could write to me and explain just exactly how it does so. Up to now, no biochemist has managed this clever trick.

I will finish this chapter by pointing out a fact that I find pertinent to the discussion. The liver is quite capable of turning one type of chemical into almost any other type of chemical. It can turn protein into sugar, sugar into fat, glycerol into glucose, etc. If you eat a great deal of carbohydrate (which is all converted into glucose), the liver will then convert excess glucose into fat. The body can only store about 2,000 calories of glucose in total, and once this limit is reached there is only thing to do with it: convert it to fat, then store it in adipose (i.e. fatty) tissue.

And what sort of fat does the liver choose to make in this situation? Super-healthy unsaturated fats? Ah, that would be a no. When the liver makes fats, it makes saturated fats, and saturated fats alone. My God, do our own livers not know how unhealthy this is? Killed by our own treacherous physiology... Or perhaps the liver knows that saturated fats are not actually unhealthy at all.

I will let you decide.

Fig. 11 Cholesterol Synthesis

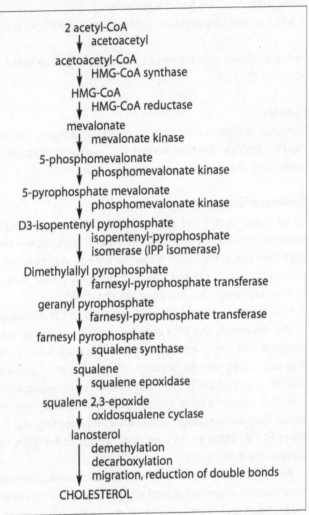

CHAPTER 3

YOU CANNOT HAVE A CHOLESTEROL LEVEL

Right, now, forget everything you have just read. (What do you mean you already have? Damn cheek.) The fact is that, after all that I have written about cholesterol and related subjects... you do not actually have a cholesterol level in your bloodstream at all.

You can read that statement again if you want to.

This fact, I believe, underpins the confusion highlighted in the letter below.

> I am 52 and recently had my first cholesterol test. When I rang the surgery for my results, the receptionist said that they were '3.3, well below the 5.5 safe maximum – and 5.5, well below the safe maximum of 7.4.' I am confused as to why I was given two numbers, and the receptionist couldn't explain. What do they mean?
> Letter in Health Section of the Independent,
> 27 September 2005

Curiouser and curiouser. Well, what could this possibly mean? Is it really possible to have two levels of the same substance in your bloodstream? Actually, nowadays, you can have at least four different cholesterol levels:

The 'good' cholesterol level

The 'bad' cholesterol level

The total cholesterol level
The ratio of 'good' to 'bad' cholesterol

And just to warn you, several more types of cholesterol level are on the way.

Ah yes, good cholesterol and bad cholesterol. A concept so mind-boggling in its stupidity that it should really have won first prize in the 'Alice in Wonderland Comes to Life in the Real World' contest. Below is a diagram of cholesterol.

Fig. 12 Cholesterol

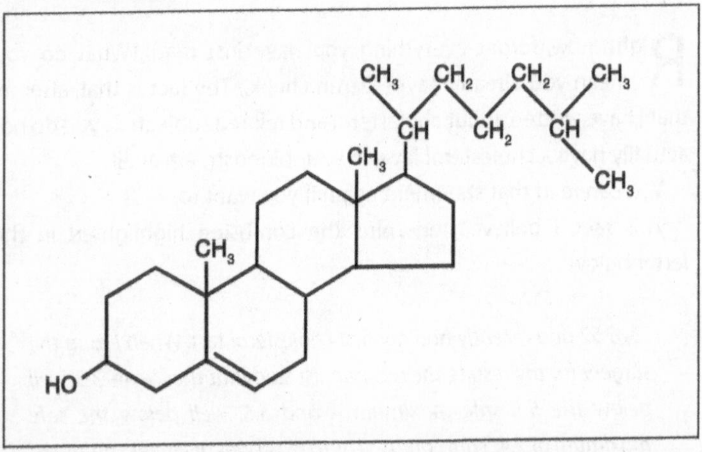

This is the only form that cholesterol comes in. It does not have right-handed 'good' cholesterol with a sinister twin called 'bad' cholesterol. So, what is all this terminology about? What does it all mean? And why can't you have a cholesterol level?

Back to basics

Cholesterol does not dissolve in water; thus, it does not dissolve in blood. This means that it has to be transported around the body inside a small transportation molecule, known as a lipoprotein (Fig.13).

Fig. 13 Lipoprotein

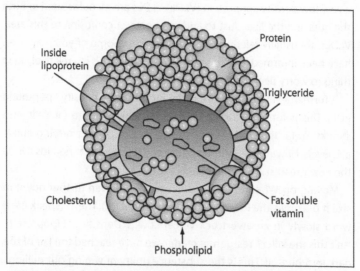

Another substance that cannot dissolve in blood is fat. So fats also travel about as part of lipoproteins. A-ha! A connection between fat and cholesterol. Yes, you're right. Fats/triglycerides and cholesterol are co-passengers inside lipoproteins. Hold that thought... then bin it – it doesn't actually go anywhere.

There are several different types of lipoprotein. The biggest is called a chylomicron, not a lipoprotein. As with almost everything in the wacky world of heart disease, the nomenclature appears to have been designed to make things difficult to follow. A chylomicron is one form of lipoprotein, but of course it isn't called a lipoprotein. That would be far too easy.

Anyway, this particular lipoprotein is manufactured in the guts. After a meal it fills up with triglyceride (fat), alongside a relatively small amount of cholesterol. The chylomicron then travels straight to fat cells in the body without passing through the liver. When the chylomicron reaches fat cells, the triglyceride is sucked out, and the chylomicron shrivels up into a little wizened remnant that is then, probably, hoovered up by the liver.

One level down in size from a chylomicron is a lipoprotein known as a very low density lipoprotein (VLDL). VLDLs are manufactured in both the guts and the liver. Just to add even greater confusion to this area, VLDLs are usually referred to as 'triglycerides'. Some of you may even have been informed as to your triglyceride level (this is a relatively new thing to worry people with).

A further level down in size is the intermediate density lipoprotein (IDL). This is formed when a VLDL loses triglyceride to fat cells, and shrinks. So far the world seems to have been spared worrying about IDL levels. However, I await the paper any day now that heralds IDL as the new, greatest danger to health.

Moving on. When the IDL shrinks to a level even further down in size it becomes the low density lipoprotein (LDL). The... (speak each word slowly in an awestruck voice) Low... Density... Lipoprotein. Isn't this the killer? Yes, gentle reader, we have reached the lair of the dark lord himself. This is the substance guilty of wiping out millions of people each and every year.

For LDL is also known 'bad' cholesterol. Even though, of course, it isn't cholesterol at all. So stop calling it cholesterol.... you idiots! Sorry, that doesn't mean you. I am ranting here at scientists, doctors and the healthcare profession in general. No wonder everyone is confused, when the terminology used is completely bonkers:

- A chylomicron is a lipoprotein, but it's never called that.
- A VLDL is a lipoprotein but it is usually called a triglyceride.
- A LDL is a lipoprotein but it is called 'bad' cholesterol.
- A high density lipoprotein (HDL), the smallest lipoprotein, is called 'good' cholesterol.

I'm a little teapot short and stout; lift me up and pour me out.

Actually, just to make things even more confusing – if that were possible – there is another form of LDL. Yes, I'm afraid so. It is exactly the same as LDL, apart from one thing. It has two types of protein attached to the outside. (All lipoproteins have proteins attached to their outer surface. This is how receptors on cells throughout the body recognise them.) This form of lipoprotein, however, is called lipoprotein(a). Good heavens, a lipoprotein that is called a lipoprotein – it must be some sort of a record. Anyway, this lipoprotein is usually pronounced as 'el pee little A' and written as Lp(a). Almost no one, including 99 per cent of doctors, knows that Lp(a) is actually LDL. Even though this fact is of fundamental importance to understanding heart disease. (More on this later.)

Why isn't Lp(a) called LDL(a), or something of the sort? Because then everyone would know what it was, and that would never do. (By the way, no one ever tells you what your Lp(a) level is. Which is typical, as it is the only one that may actually be important.)

I have just realised that I have been remiss in not mentioning high density lipoproteins, or HDL, or 'good' cholesterol. This lipoprotein, it is thought, is mainly manufactured in the liver. ('What do you mean 'thought,' surely all this stuff is known?' Sorry, no it's not.) Anyway, it is believed that HDL 'removes' cholesterol from plaques in arteries and transports it back to the liver for reprocessing. So HDL protects you from heart disease and is therefore 'good'. Even if it is not cholesterol, and, pound for pound, contains more cholesterol than any other sort of lipoprotein in the body.

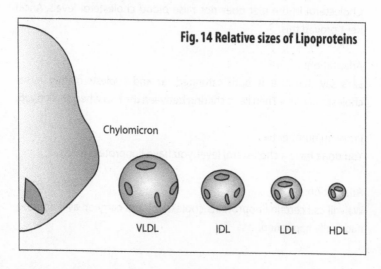

Fig. 14 Relative sizes of Lipoproteins

Chylomicron

VLDL   IDL   LDL   HDL

Frankly, the idea that an inanimate molecule can suck cholesterol out of a plaque is so laughable that I can't begin to explain here how preposterous an idea it is. And moreover, I would challenge any scientist anywhere to explain exactly how it happens. A molecule that travels both ways through a concentration gradient? 'Of course it does, now run away and play with your friends and leave the adults alone.'

The million-dollar question

As I hope I have now made abundantly clear, you do not – indeed, cannot – have a cholesterol level in your blood. So, what happened to the cholesterol hypothesis? Where'd it go? Well, although it has changed almost completely from its first incarnation, somehow or other it has also managed to remain the same.

The cholesterol hypothesis started out as something pure and simple: 'If you eat too much cholesterol, the level of cholesterol in the blood rises. Cholesterol is then deposited on artery walls causing them to thicken and narrow.' But it sure as hell hasn't stayed that way:

Problem number one:
Cholesterol in the diet does not raise blood cholesterol levels. Ancel Keys proved this.

Adaptation:
Let's say that is it is both saturated fat and cholesterol that raises cholesterol levels. Then keep shifting between the two when challenged.

Problem number two:
You don't have a cholesterol level, you have lipoprotein levels.

Adaptation:
We will call certain lipoproteins 'cholesterol' and carry on as if nothing had really happened.

'Four legs good, two legs bad' has become 'Four legs good, two legs better.' And, as George Orwell predicted, no one noticed.

Up to this point I have actually highlighted only the first two major adaptations to the cholesterol hypothesis. But over the years there has been adaptation after adaptation after adaptation. One of the more convoluted adaptations (following some horribly contradictory evidence against saturated fat causing heart disease) was that it is not saturated fat in the diet that matters, it is the ratio of polyunsaturated to saturated fat that is really important. Then it changed again, and a lack of monounsaturated fats seemed to be the critical factor. Then... well, who knows. It's tough keeping track.

Indeed, the closer you look, the more you find that the cholesterol hypothesis is a truly amazing beast. It is in a process of constant adaptation in order to encompass all contradictory data without keeling over and expiring. I sometimes think of it like a monster from a 1950s horror movie – *The Thing*, or *The Blob*. Every time you think you have killed it, it just gets back up and carries on. 'My God Chuck, attacking it with electricity has just made it stronger!'

My view is that any hypothesis that has to keep changing all the time to survive the relentless assault of contradictory facts is, in reality, a dead hypothesis. To quote James Black from a 200-year-old lecture:

> *A nice adaptation of conditions will make almost any hypothesis agree with the phenomena. This will please the imagination, but does not advance our knowledge.*
>
> J Black, *Lectures of the Elements of Chemistry, 1803*

Clever chap, James Black.

However, having an endlessly adaptable hypothesis does provide a major challenge to me. If I attack it, I will be informed that I have just attacked something that doesn't exist: 'Why are you bothered about fat intake? You should know that the real problem is a lack of Omega 3 fatty acids, and/or plant stanols, and/or antioxidants, and/or monounsaturated fats... Of course saturated fats are important, but you must consider the other important factors in conjunction. Heart disease, you see, is very much a multifactorial disease.'

If anyone ever tells me that heart disease is multifactorial again, I shall scream. It is the ultimate cop-out statement. It allows anyone to say anything, without bothering with the tiresome problem of thinking first: 'All diseases are multifactorial in some way, so let's give up trying to look for causes.' I think not.

So, at the considerable risk of zeroing in on a moving target, I will state that, as of today, the most widely accepted version of the new, improved (yet – somehow – still the original) cholesterol hypothesis is as follows:

Eating excess saturated fat in the diet raises LDL levels. The LDL, otherwise known as 'bad' cholesterol, then causes thickening and narrowing in the arteries.

Which is not really a cholesterol hypothesis, but it is still a 'diet-heart hypothesis' I guess, and perhaps it could even be true. If it is true, though, how does it actually work? How does saturated fat raise LDL levels? A primary requirement of any half-decent hypothesis in medicine is that it is biological plausible – i.e. there should be some understandable, and seemingly reasonable, underlying mechanism of action.

It must be admitted that the original idea, which was that cholesterol in the diet increased cholesterol levels, at least had the advantage of superficial plausibility. Even if, when you get down to studying it in any detail, it is revealed as total baloney. But where is the link between eating saturated fat and raising LDL levels?

As I have already explained, most of the fat in the diet – saturated or otherwise – is transported directly to fat cells, travelling inside chylomicrons. No impact on LDL there. Fat that does manage to reach the liver has zero impact on cholesterol production too. So, I will ask again: how does saturated fat (or any other type of fat, come to that) raise LDL levels?

Well, moving a step back, surely we must look at where LDL comes from? After all, LDL is what remains of a VLDL after it has shrunk in size by losing fats. VLDLs are made in the liver and are used to transport both fat and cholesterol out of the liver, and deliver both substances to cells around the body*. So, if we want to know what raises LDL levels, we surely have to ask what raises VLDL levels in the first place, as this is the one and only source of LDL. A-ha! I can almost hear you thinking: saturated fat consumption must raise the VLDL levels. Yes?

No. The thing that raises VLDL levels is eating carbohydrates... On the other hand, a high-fat diet lowers VLDL levels. Here is one more guilty little secret of heart-disease researchers exposed.

You don't believe me? Then perhaps you'll believe the American Journal of Medicine. Spurred on by a desire to prove that the Atkins diet (high fat, low carb) was dangerous, researchers fed a group of obese people an Atkins-type diet. Here are the highlights:

> PURPOSE: To compare the effects of a low-carbohydrate diet and a conventional (fat- and calorie-restricted) diet on lipoprotein subfractions and inflammation in severely obese subjects.
>
> RESULTS: Subjects on a low-carbohydrate [i.e., high-fat] diet experienced a **greater decrease** [my emphasis] in large very low-density lipoprotein [VLDL] levels.[4]

And subsequently, a bigger study presented at the American Heart Association demonstrated the following:

> In the most recent study, presented at the annual scientific meeting of the American Heart Association in Chicago, Duke

---

* (Pedantic point) The VLDL that is made in the guts does not become LDL, so for the purposes of this discussion we can ignore it. The reason why it doesn't become LDL is that VLDL made in the gut has a different type of protein attached to it, so although it does shrink in size, it is not recognised by LDL receptors. If you really want to know the detail, gut-derived VLDL has apolipoprotein B-48 attached to it. Liver-derived VLDL has apolipoprotein B-100 attached to it. It is the B-100 apolipoprotein that locks into an LDL receptor, at which point the entire LDL is pulled into the cell and broken down into its component parts.

4 Seshadri, P, Iqbal, N, Stern, L, Williams, M, Chicano, KL, Daily, DA, McGrory, J, Gracely, EJ, Rader, DJ, Samaha, FF. 'A Randomized Study Comparing the Effects of a Low-Carbohydrate Diet and a Conventional Diet on Lipoprotein Subfractions and C-Reactive Protein Levels in Patients with Severe Obesity', American Journal of Medicine, 117(5), 2004, pages 398–405.

University researchers randomly assigned 120 overweight volunteers to the Atkins diet or to the American Heart Association's low-fat 'Step I' diet. People on the Atkins diet restricted their carbohydrate intake to less than 20 grams a day, with 60 percent of their calories coming from fat.

After six months, participants on the Atkins diet had lost 31 pounds, had an 11 percent increase in HDL [i.e., 'good' cholesterol] and a 49 percent [my emphasis] drop in their triglyceride [VLDL] levels.'

http://www.thyroid-info.com/dietnews/11nov.htm#atkins

Here you have it, then. VLDL is the only source of LDL, but when you eat more fat the VLDL level drops. In one study it dropped by very nearly 50 per cent. This should mean that eating fat will, in turn, lower LDL levels, shouldn't it? Well, actually it doesn't. A high-fat diet neither raises nor lowers LDL levels.

How can this be? If VLDL is the only source of LDL then if you have more VLDL to start with, you must end up with more LDL in the bloodstream in the end, surely? Help, what on earth is going on?

It's time for the final twist in this particular saga: there is absolutely no connection whatsoever between the VLDL level and the LDL level. It has been known for a long time that over a period of days – even weeks, months and usually years – the LDL level remains fixed – no matter what you eat. And no matter what happens to the VLDL level. LDL levels can rise and fall, true, but in the majority of people this only happens gradually, and certainly not within a 24-hour period. In short, the VLDL level can shoot up and down while the LDL level remains locked.

And what does this tell us, exactly? It tells us that LDL can be removed at whatever rate is needed to keep LDL levels constant, no matter how much VLDL shrinks down to become LDL. Also, that the system controlling LDL levels is unaffected by what you eat, or the amount of VLDL manufactured by the liver. All of this, by the way, is known by researchers who specialise in lipids. And now you know it too.

However, it rather begs the question: if they know all this, what is their explanation as to how saturated fat raises LDL levels? I would ask you to have a guess, but there is no way on earth you would be able to come up with the current, preposterous, conjecture. For it is this:

> If you eat saturated fat, this will reduce the number of LDL receptors – the things that lock on to LDL and pull it out of the bloodstream – thus causing the LDL level to rise.

Why would eating saturated fat do this? There is no connection between saturated-fat consumption and the needs of cells around the body to absorb LDL – none. You might as well suggest that eating protein causes your hair to grow faster. It makes as much sense.

Perhaps you think that this is all theoretical, and doesn't matter at all. 'Surely it must have been proven by now that saturated fat does cause LDL levels to rise, so forget the clever arguments, Dr Kendrick.' In fact this has never been proven. Or, to be more accurate, some studies have shown a rise, some a fall. Others have shown nothing at all. I will mention some of these later. [5]

For now, I will stick to one quote from the Framingham Study which is the most influential, longest-running, and most oft-quoted study in heart-disease research. It began in 1948, and it is still running today, which also makes it the longest study that has ever been done.

> *In Framingham, Massachusetts, the more saturated fat one ate, the more cholesterol one ate, the more calories one ate, the lower people's serum cholesterol [by which he means LDL – my note].*
>
> Dr William Castelli, Director of the Framingham Study, 1992

When I show this quote to other doctors it makes them choke on their tea. But it shouldn't. How can eating saturated fat raise LDL levels? It is

5 http://www.jaoa.org/cgi/reprint/102/7/377 This shows no change in LDL levels on an AHA Step One diet. Some went up, some went down, most stayed the same.

not merely biologically implausible, it is biologically impossible. It always was, and it always will be. (Boy, does that statement make me a hostage to fortune!)

AND FINALLY...

Before moving on from this area, I thought I should give you a quick rundown on the different cholesterol levels that you hear about nowadays, and what they are thought to represent.

Total cholesterol

This is still, probably, the most common figure given out to patients. The total cholesterol level is reached by adding together levels of the 'evil' LDL, plus the 'saintly' HDL, plus a few other wayward lipoproteins – IDL and suchlike – that get mixed up in the analysis. (You think that cholesterol level is a super-accurate measurement? Ho, ho.)

The average total cholesterol level in the UK is about 6.1 – expressed as mmol/l (millimoles per litre). Anything above 7mmol/l and your GP will send for the local priest to read out the last rites. At present, the figure that the healthcare profession aims to achieve, through statination, is about 5.0mmol/l. Oh we do like a nice round figure, it's so neat and tidy and scientific – not.

'Good' cholesterol

This is the high density lipoprotein level (HDL), which normally sits at about 1.3mmol/l. Anything below 0.9mmol/l and your life-insurance company will cancel your subscription, then paint a little black spot in the middle of your palm for good luck. Above 2.0mmol/l, and you can get the Saga booklets out and look forward to a long and happy career in lawn-green bowling.

'Bad' cholesterol level

This is the low density lipoprotein (LDL) level. On average, this is about 3.5mmol/l. Anything above 4mmol/l and you will be statinated. Resistance is useless.

The ratio of good to bad cholesterol

Clearly, if HDL is good and LDL is bad, you could have a high total cholesterol level yet still be 'healthy'. If, that is, your total cholesterol level is boosted by a high HDL. So some people think that what's really important is the ratio of good to bad cholesterol. I shall remain silent on this point, because I was taught that if you can think of nothing nice to say, you should say nothing at all.

One rather critical point about cholesterol levels that I have not mentioned so far is that the level which is considered high has been falling relentlessly. Twenty years ago, GPs in the UK would only get excited if your total cholesterol level was above about 7.0mmol/l. Ten years ago, anything above 6.5mmol/l had moved into the 'treatment' zone. Today, if your level is above 5.0mmol/l you will be earmarked for 'statination'. Tomorrow, if current trends continue, the level will be 4.0mmol/l. It already is for those who have suffered a heart attack. Some 'experts' believe that the true, healthy level of cholesterol is about 2.5mmol/l. Therefore, no matter what your level of cholesterol, according to the prevailing wisdom, you will benefit from having it lowered.

Here is a short section from an article by Law and Wald in the British Medical Journal (BMJ) from 2002. They argue that the levels of both cholesterol (and blood pressure) in all westernised societies are far higher than those of our ancestors and the remaining hunter-gatherer populations dotted around the world. In their opinion, therefore, limiting statin treatment to people with a total blood cholesterol of 4.0mmol/l, or even 3.0mmol/l, is actively dangerous.

> ... *everyone needs blood pressure, and cholesterol is essential for life. These lower limits are, however, beyond Western values and not reached by current dietary or drug interventions. They should not be invoked as obstacles to offering effective preventive treatments.*
> *http://bmj.bmjjournals.com/cgi/content/full/324/7353/1570*

Translation: everyone in the UK should take statins now, and for the rest their lives. You may have heard of Law and Wald before, via their Polypill concept. A concept that – were the Polypill to take off – would make Law and Wald rich beyond the dreams of Croesus. Yes, these were the authors of that piece.

Moving on, here is a section from the BBC's website, reporting on a conference on the wider use of statins:

> *Dr John Reckless, chairman of Heart UK and a consultant endocrinologist at Bath University, put forward the case.*
>
> *'The whole point of the debate is to bring out the fact that we are under-treating and the fact that a lot more people could benefit.*
>
> *'The whole population should be following diet, lifestyle and weight loss measures. We shouldn't have our high-fat meals and we shouldn't lounge around, we should all be taking exercise and so on.*
>
> *'Of course we all need that. But on the other hand, rather more people do need statins than are currently getting them.*
>
> *'So maybe people should be able to have their statin, perhaps if not in their drinking water, with their drinking water.'*
>
> http://news.bbc.co.uk/2/hi/health/3931157.stm

Statins in the drinking water?

CHAPTER 4

WHAT ARE STATINS AND HOW DO THEY WORK?

> One of the first duties of the physician is to
> educate the masses not to take medicine.
> Sir William Osler, MD (1849-1919)

There are a number of different statins:

- Lovastatin
- Fluvastatin
- Pravastatin
- Simvastatin
- Cerivastatin
- Atorvastatin
- Rosuvastatin

Why so many? Actually, as mentioned before, cerivastatin was voluntarily withdrawn after killing rather too many people. Somewhat inconveniently, it was said to cause muscle disintegration, followed by death. (In fact, all statins can cause muscle disintegration and death, although the risk seems to be greatest with cerivastatin.) So at least you can cross cerivastatin off your list. Which leaves a mere six in active service. In my opinion, that's six too many.

Statins all come under different brand names in different countries. In the UK, the only one that is available over the counter (OTC) – thus not requiring a doctor's prescription – is simvastatin. This is also known as Zocor, or Zocor Heart Pro. Which should be said in a kind of awestruck American/Hollywood film announcer-type accent. You know the sort of thing:

'He was a man with heart disease.

'She was a doctor with a passion for saving lives.

'Together, they discovered Zocor Heart Pro... and nothing would ever be the same again...'

Atorvastatin (Lipitor), and simvastatin (Zocor), are among the most widely prescribed of the statins. Lipitor sits proudly at the top of the sales pyramid with over £6 billion per year in sales worldwide. Rosuvastatin (Crestor) was the latest to hit the market. It was discovered in Japan, and the marketing rights were sold to AstraZeneca. It has not done as well as was hoped.

All statins are also known as HMG-CoA Reductase Inhibitors – because inhibiting the actions of the enzyme known as HMG-CoA reductase is what they actually do. If you remember my horribly complicated diagram of cholesterol synthesis from earlier on, one of the steps is the following:

Fig. 15 Where statins work

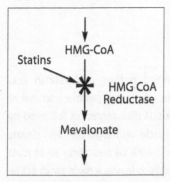

I think that this diagram (Fig. 15) represents about step four in the long and winding road from converting Acetyl CoA to cholesterol.

And why, you might ask, have scientists not found ways to inhibit other steps in cholesterol synthesis? Why this particular one? It is not for a want of trying, that's for sure. However, problems ensued with drugs that acted elsewhere in cholesterol synthesis – problems such as the death of the surrounding organism, for example. This was a fairly common problem and tended to negate the huge health benefits gained from reduced cholesterol production...

A conundrum

Now, those who were paying attention earlier on may just have spotted a problem with how statins work. If not, I will point it out to you anyway:

- Statins reduce the synthesis of cholesterol. (Yes.)
- By reducing cholesterol synthesis, they should in turn reduce the production of VLDL in the liver. (Yes.)
- VLDLs shrink to form LDLs. (Yes.)
- So, if you have fewer VLDLs, the level of LDL will drop. (Ah. No.)

As explained in the last chapter, there is no association between the VLDL level and the LDL level, so that's not the answer. Or, at least, that's far from the whole answer. In fact, the LDL level is controlled by the number of LDL receptors in the body. The more LDL receptors you have, the more LDL will be removed from the circulation.

Unlike VLDL, or IDL, LDLs do not shrink, thereby changing into other types of lipoprotein. LDLs wander about in the circulation, essentially unaltered, until they lock on to an LDL receptor. At this point, the LDL and all of its contents are pulled into cells and then broken down, along with the receptor itself. So if you have a million LDL receptors waving about trying to attract some passing LDL, a million LDLs will be removed from the circulation. And if you want to remove more LDLs, more receptors must be manufactured, then transported to the surface of the cell – wherever in the body those cells may be.

At this point, I think it would be timely to mention a condition by the name of Familial Hypercholesterolaemia (FH), in which LDL levels are extremely high. In some cases, levels are more than five times 'normal'. The underlying problem in FH is a lack of LDL receptors. With very few receptors available, LDL is stuck in the circulation and consequently its level skyrockets. The LDL receptor – or lack of it in FH – was discovered by two scientists called Brown and Goldstein in 1973. For their work in this area they were awarded the Nobel prize.

* * * * *

OK, time out for a second. By now you may well find that your head is swimming with facts and stats. I did say that this stuff was a bit complicated. I also realise that you may be thinking to yourself:'Boring! who needs to know this?' You need to know this, I believe, because you need to know that the entire cholesterol/diet-heart hypothesis is nothing like you thought it was. Nor are statins super-simple things that lower so-called 'cholesterol levels' through the simple mechanism of reducing cholesterol production in the liver.

In fact, I often think that if those who started the whole cholesterol shebang had any idea how damn complicated it would all turn out to be, once they started thinking it through, they would have realised that it couldn't possibly work. But they didn't. They kept clinging to cholesterol while all else crumbled around them. I think it's a kind of quasi-religious thing:'We cannot lose faith…'

What I do find somewhat ironic is that statins were designed to reduce cholesterol production in the liver, thus lowering cholesterol levels. And this is exactly what they do! This is despite the fact that you don't actually have a cholesterol level in the blood in the first place. How strange is that? Very, actually. It's so strange that I can't even think of a suitable analogy.

In a nutshell, statins work (to lower cholesterol levels) in the following way:

1: They lower cholesterol synthesis in the liver.
2: The liver starts running out of the cholesterol needed to make VLDLs.
3: The liver then has to increase the number of LDL receptors to pull cholesterol back in to make more VLDLs.
4: More LDL is dragged back into the liver, as a result of which…
5: The LDL level in the blood falls.
So now you know. Very simple really.

Other actions of statins

But if you think that the only action of statins is to reduce the synthesis of cholesterol in the liver, then you are very much mistaken. Statins do many other things. Drugs are very rarely like Koch's 'magic bullets' of yore, designed to pick off one precise bacterium, or enzyme, or biochemical action, in the body.

With most drugs, putting them into the body is a bit like handing a five-year-old an Uzi 9mm machine gun in a hostage situation, then hoping that when the ammo runs out the net result will be that more bad guys got killed than good guys. Sometimes yes, sometimes no. Take steroids, for example. This is a class of drugs that act just about everywhere in the body, and they can be used to treat a huge range of different conditions. For example:

- Eczema
- Organ transplantation – to prevent rejection
- Rheumatoid arthritis
- Ulcerative colitis
- Asthma
- Injection into tennis elbow
- Inability to win a gold medal at the Olympics

How precise is that? Not very.

And how about thalidomide – designed initially as a sedative to treat morning sickness, but found to create terrible limb deformities in babies? However, the very action that stops limbs from forming properly in unborn children also stops tumours growing by preventing the formation of new blood vessels. Currently, thalidomide is the hottest new thing in cancer treatment.

Or Viagra. Developed to treat angina, found to create long-lasting erections by the students enrolled in clinical studies. And no, they didn't get many unused Viagra tablets back. Interestingly, Viagra may now have come full circle as it is increasingly being used to treat pulmonary hypertension (high blood pressure in the lungs).

Finally, and perhaps most pertinent to this discussion, is the drug aspirin. Aspirin started life as a painkiller – mainly. About 40 years ago, it was found to 'thin' the blood by stopping platelets sticking together.

Consequently, aspirin is now used to prevent heart attacks. Who would ever have guessed?

In short, drugs almost always have a wide range of different actions. Some expected, some completely unexpected. And statins are no exception to this rule. Thus, it is fully possible that statins may have 'coincidental' effects on preventing heart disease that have nothing whatsoever to do with lowering LDL levels.

You think I am stretching things a bit here? Then read this:

> There is increasing evidence, however, that statins may also exert effects beyond cholesterol lowering. Indeed, many of these cholesterol-independent or 'pleiotropic' vascular effects of statins appear to involve restoring or improving endothelial function through increasing the bioavailability of nitric oxide, promoting re-endothelialization, reducing oxidative stress, and inhibiting inflammatory responses. Thus, the endothelium-dependent effects of statins are thought to contribute to many of the beneficial effects of statin therapy in cardiovascular disease.
>
> http://atvb.ahajournals.org/cgi/content/full/23/5/729

Too much scientific gobbledegook? Sorry, but it does make the point that statins have a whole series of effects on blood vessels that could be protective against heart disease. At the last count I got together 35 'non-cholesterol-lowering' actions of statins.

You're still doubtful? Well, I hope to convince you later on that the 'non-cholesterol-lowering' actions of statins are – in fact – the only possible explanation as to how they work. After all, there were plenty of drugs around that lowered cholesterol before statins were discovered. But only statins showed any significant benefit in treating cardiovascular disease. And why would this be, I wonder?

CHAPTER 5

THE RISE AND RISE OF THE CHOLESTEROL HYPOTHESIS

B efore starting on the Herculean task of destroying the entire cholesterol hypothesis, I thought it would be interesting to look at how, and why, it developed in the first place. And then how it went on to take over the world.

Shockingly, I have found that it was a huge conspiracy between right-wing governments across the world, pursuing a neo-imperialist pro-globalisation agenda, in conjunction with the pharmaceutical industry!

Oh, OK, so it wasn't. It was more a case of people under huge pressure to come up with answers grasping the wrong end of stick, then seeing exactly what they wanted to see, and ignoring all evidence to the contrary. To quote Bing Crosby: 'You've got to acc-entuate the positive, e-liminate the negative.' Which, speaking as a 'negative', is slightly worrying. Perhaps I will end up as part of the foundations for a huge new statin-manufacturing plant…

To find out how the cholesterol hypothesis actually started, we have to travel back far into the past, to Berlin in the mid-19th century. Let us peer into the laboratory of a brilliant and already famous pathologist, Rudolf Von Virchow. Although it's late at night young Rudolf is still working, his mind ever active. He is gazing with feverish intent through a powerful new microscope at the arteries of corpses (though they were not necessarily all the victims of heart disease). He has noted that the arteries have thickened 'plaques' in them, and he wants to know more.

And tonight he makes a breakthrough discovery that will echo throughout history for the next 150 years. He has found that the plaques in the arteries contain a great deal of cholesterol. And where, he ponders, could this cholesterol have come from? The blood seems the only possible place. In a state of agitation, he jumps up, leaps upon his horse and gallops through the streets of Berlin shouting 'Eureka'. (Actually, perhaps that was someone else…)

The thing about this (admittedly over-dramatised) story that I am most impressed by is that Virchow was able to recognise cholesterol when he saw it. However, despite Virchow's findings, very little actually moved forward during his lifetime. His was an era in which medicine was preoccupied with infectious diseases. In 1850 you could still die from a small scratch. Tuberculosis felled millions, as did infection during childbirth. Anyone who managed to avoid an infectious death and ended up clutching their chest from a heart attack was probably considered to have done pretty well. 'A heart attack, young man, is the sign of a long life, well-lived.' (Actually, no one would have said this, because no one knew what a heart attack was back then: it was called discombubulitis praecordia, and considered – by learned opinion leaders of the time – to be due to a lack of prompt leech application.)

Thus many years passed without anyone taking much interest in heart disease. Indeed, it would seem to have been at least 50 years before the next significant move forward was made, this time by Dr Nikolai Anitschkov, a Russian researcher. He fed rabbits a high-cholesterol diet; their arteries then thickened and filled up with cholesterol. So, cholesterol in the diet is deadly, and causes heart disease in humans – case proven? Well, Anitschkov certainly thought so.

And how silly of me even to question such research. Let me see. Rabbits are carnivores… check. Rabbits normally eat a high-cholesterol diet… check. And the thickenings that they get in their arteries are exactly the same as those found in humans… check. Ergo, feeding rabbits is an excellent model for heart-disease causation in humans… check.

Perhaps Anitschkov should have fed cats the normal diet of a rabbit, just to see how long they would have lasted. I would give it a week, max. Frankly, trying to prove anything about humans by carrying out dietary experiments on rabbits is nonsense. But when your aim is to push a cholesterol hypothesis, such results look good, and appear superficially convincing. As do many things if you avoid thinking about them too hard.

If you add Anitschkov to Virchow, the cholesterol bandwagon had started to roll. As no one else had any particularly strong opinions on the matter at this time – at least, none that I have come across – the putative diet-heart/cholesterol hypothesis established itself in the number-one position as the cause of heart disease, and has remained at the top of the heap ever since, swatting all pretenders effortlessly into touch.

However, even after Anitschkov, no one was really that interested in heart disease. Was this because it was very rare, or not recognised? Hard to say. The first medical description of a heart attack was not published until 1926 by Dr James B Herrick, in the USA. Even then, I get the impression that this was seen as a medical rarity, not something to get the entire medical community excited.

In reality, it was not until after WWII that doctors started to get really interested in heart disease. After the upheaval of the war was over, people noticed that middle-aged men were dropping like flies. This appeared to be the start of an 'epidemic' that had swept in from nowhere, and it began in the USA.

Or did it? One thing that I have discovered during my trawls back through the history of heart disease is how much of the information is less than reliable. For example, it wasn't until a few years after WWII that the World Health Organization (WHO) got its act together and created an International Classification of Diseases (ICD). Prior to this, different countries had different ways of classifying disease. Some countries had diseases that didn't exist in others, and vice versa. Heart disease was a big mess, and it is almost impossible to work out who was classifying what, as what, or why. France, for example, did not move to using full ICD classification until 1968. And the French had no term for a myocardial infarction until this time.

So, it is fully possible that heart disease, or coronary heart disease (CHD), was wiping out millions in the 1930s, but that no one really noticed. I have to admit that this sounds unlikely, but the ability of doctors to ignore diseases that they haven't been trained to recognise is a recurrent pattern in medicine. 'It's not in a textbook, so it doesn't exist. Now, pray be silent on the matter.'

My own view – which, admittedly, I cannot fully support – is that heart disease (of the sort this book is interested in) was at quite a high level in the USA in the 1920s and 1930s, but went unnoticed. The upheaval of WWII obscured a further rise in the 1940s, and the true extent of heart disease only really came to light after this.

Fig. 16 USA death rates for major cardiovascular diseases 1900-1997
(Exhibit A)

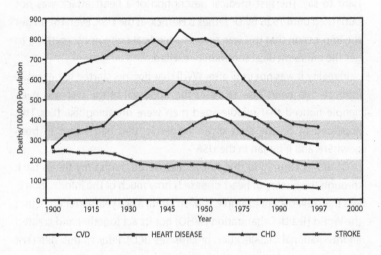

In support of my argument, I produce exhibit A (Fig 16). This is a graph of death rates for major cardiovascular diseases in the USA from 1900 to 1997. May I draw your attention to a number of features in particular:

1: CHD did not exist until 1948, when the WHO decided that it did. So there are no deaths from CHD before that, but plenty afterwards.

2: There is a rapid rise in CHD from 1948 until about 1965, or thereabouts, then a fall for the next 30 years. However, this is completely out of synch with the level of 'heart disease', which peaked in about 1948 and has fallen ever since.

3: The total number of cardiovascular deaths (CVD) – which is the combination of all heart disease and strokes – also peaked in about 1948, then fell.

4: From about 1940 to 1965, the rate of death from 'heart disease' remained relatively constant, although the rate of CHD rose sharply during this period.

5: From about 1965, the rate of death from CVD, 'heart disease' and CHD run almost parallel, in contrast to the previous 20 years.

I think that there is only one possible interpretation of these figures, which is that it took around 20 years for many doctors to start using the new 'disease' classification of coronary heart disease (CHD) properly. Until 1965, therefore, a number of deaths from CHD were being misclassified under the generic term 'heart disease'.

What this almost certainly means is that the peak of deaths from CHD in the USA occurred before 1965, possibly in 1948 itself. You won't read that in any textbook, but it's probably true. Therefore, if you can assume – as I think you can – that many people who died of 'heart disease' prior to 1948 were really dying from CHD, then it would appear likely that CHD was actually killing people in large numbers in the 1920s and 1930s.

Is this important? It may be, for reasons that I hope to explain a bit later on. But I think this example mainly highlights the fact that you have to be extremely careful in interpreting medical data, and not take it too literally. If you did, you could end up making a statement such as the following: 'CHD did not exist in the USA until 1948. At which point it suddenly started killing millions of people. It rose to a peak in 1965, and has fallen since.' That is, literally, what the previous graph indicates. But it clearly doesn't represent the true picture. What can be said about CHD in the USA, I believe, is that it (probably) rose rapidly during the 1920s and 1930s, peaked some time between 1948 and 1965, and has fallen ever since.

Over the next 50 years, a number of different populations have taken over the USA's mantle as holder of the 'top death rate from heart disease'.

Heart disease – the top six

1950s – USA
1960s – Finland
1970s – Scotland
1980s – Poland
1990s – Rest of eastern Europe
2000s – Emigrant Asian Indians/Aboriginals in Australia and North America

---

More about these populations later. However, in this particular historical trawl I was most interested to establish the point when the diet-heart hypothesis became the number-one hypothesis. That said, spotting the point at which an idea achieves dominance is tricky. Often ideas seem to have been around forever, and it is surprising to find how recent they are.

For example: tectonic plate movement. First proposed in 1912 by Alfred Wegener, immediately followed by harsh ridicule. Dr Rollin T Chamberlin of the University of Chicago commented, 'Wegener's hypothesis in general is of the footloose type, in that it takes considerable liberty with our globe, and is less bound by restrictions or tied down by awkward, ugly facts than most of its rival theories.' The concept of tectonic plate movement was stomped on with pitiless hostility for the next 50 years or so, then accepted as self-evident truth in about 1965, or thereabouts. Rather more recently than you thought, I would guess.

And with heart disease, despite Virchow and Anitshkof and Herrick and others, it is clear that the diet-heart hypothesis was not remotely dominant until well after WWII. Below is a passage describing a seminal meeting in the 1950s that demonstrates this fact nicely. It was written by Henry Blackburn, a friend and supporter of Ancel Keys. Here he discusses his view on the motivation of Ancel Keys to carry out his huge dietary studies:

> In 1954, the fledgling World Health Organization called its first Expert Committee on the Pathogenesis of Atherosclerosis to consider the burgeoning epidemic of coronary disease and heart attacks. Several medical leaders of the time were assembled in Geneva: Paul Dudley White of Boston, Gunnar Björk of Stockholm, Noboru Kimura of Japan, George Pickering of Oxford, Ancel Keys of Minnesota, and others. As reported by Pickering the discussion was lively, tending to tangents and tirades.
>
> Ancel Keys was in good form – outspoken, quick, typically blunt. When at this critical conference, he posed with such assurance his dietary hypothesis of coronary heart disease, he was ill prepared for the indignant reaction of some.
>
> George Pickering, recently named Knight of the Realm by Queen Elizabeth, interrupted Keys' peroration. He put it something along these lines: 'Tell us, Professor Keys, if you would be so kind, what is the single best piece of evidence you can cite in support of your thesis about diet and coronary heart disease?
>
> Keys, ordinarily quick on the draw, was taken aback. Rarely, of course, is there ever a 'single best piece of evidence' supporting any

theory. Theory is developed from a body of evidence and varied sources. This is particularly true in regard to the many facts of lifestyle that relate to disease. It is the totality and congruity of evidence that leads to a theory – and to inference of causation.

Keys fell headlong into the trap. He proceeded to cite a piece of evidence. Sir George and the assembled peers were easily able to diminish this single piece of evidence, and did so. And by then it was too late to recover – for Keys to summon the total evidence in a constructive, convincing argument.

My theory is that Keys was so stung by this event that he left the Geneva meeting intent on gathering the definitive evidence to establish or refute the Diet-Heart theory. Out of this single, moving, personal experience – so my theory goes – came the challenge, the motivation, and eventually, the implementation of the Seven Countries Study.

http://www.epi.umn.edu/about/7countries/index.shtm

So there you have it. As a result, Ancel Keys stormed off, put together a huge research budget, hired a staff of thousands, did his study and was then able – in objective 'scientific speak', of course – to go 'I told you so, I told you so. Nyah, nyah, nyah!'

However, Keys's supporter Henry Blackburn, claimed, 'Oh, the study has been criticised for the method in which populations were selected.'

Before getting pulled too far off track, let me summarise my main points:

1: It was not until some time in the early 1950s that coronary heart disease (CHD) was seen as a massive health problem. Recognition first occurred in the USA, almost certainly because the USA did have by far the highest rate of heart disease at that time…

2: At this point panic ensued. Stung into action, the medical profession needed some answers – fast. Mainly the answers to two rather important questions.

- What causes heart disease?
- How do we prevent it, or cure it?

Suddenly the earlier work of Virchow and Anitschkov became relevant. A Russian researcher called Kritchevsky carried out experiments on rabbits, published his work and was hailed as a hero. Cometh the hour, cometh the research study.

But the main man was Ancel Keys, and his famous Seven Countries Study. Keys looked at saturated-fat consumption in seven countries and found a straight-line relationship between heart disease, cholesterol levels and saturated-fat intake. The seven countries were:

- Italy
- Greece
- Former Yugoslavia
- Netherlands
- Finland
- USA
- Japan

Why these particular seven countries? He could have chosen another seven and demonstrated the exact opposite. Here are my seven countries:

- Finland
- Israel
- Netherlands
- Germany
- Switzerland
- France
- Sweden

What do you mean I can't choose my own countries? That's not fair. Keys did.

Despite the crippling flaws of his study. Most people believed that Keys had proven the diet-heart hypothesis beyond doubt. At which point the evidence seemed to flood in from all over the place. In 1948 – a good year for heart disease – a study had been set up in the town of Framingham, near Boston. The whole population was screened for 'factors' that might be involved in causing heart disease, and then studied for years and years. In fact, the study continues today – which, for some reason, I find a bit creepy.

One of the first findings to emerge from the Framingham Study during the 1950s was that the level of cholesterol in the blood was the best predictor of the chance of dying of CHD. So another piece of the jigsaw slipped into place. It wasn't just rabbits who died of high blood-cholesterol levels. Humans did too.

Other researchers looking further back in time noted that rationing was introduced during WWII in Norway and the UK, and in both countries the rate of heart disease fell. (Although the rate of having bombs fall on your head rose rapidly, which could have had something to do with a rapid alteration in the causes of death.)

It was then found that there were some people with a genetic condition known as familial hypercholesterolaemia (FH) – basically, an inherited condition of high levels of blood cholesterol (LDL). Children inheriting the condition from both parents could die as young as five from heart disease. By golly, it was all beginning to look like an open-and-shut case.

Leaping ahead in time somewhat; in the 1970s Brown and Goldstein identified that people with FH had a problem with their production of LDL receptors. With fewer LDL receptors the LDL level skyrocketed and this was the basic 'fault' in FH – which, as you will now recognise, should actually be called 'hyper low density lipoproteinemia.' It was at this time that the concept of a raised blood cholesterol started to fragment into a constellation of different lipoproteins, and LDL was fingered as 'bad' cholesterol.

And so it seemed – although I am leaping about a bit in time and space – that all the pieces of the jigsaw puzzle were falling into place and the diet-heart hypothesis was really flying. As early as 1956 the American Heart Association (AHA), somewhat jumping the gun in my opinion, had launched the concept of the 'prudent diet'. A prudent diet consisted of replacing butter with margarine, beef with skinless chicken, bacon and eggs with cold cereal, warm baths with cold showers and chocolate by a smack on the back of the neck with a cold kipper.

In the 1960s and 1970s, huge trials on dietary modification were set up. The biggest was probably the MR-FIT trial, involving hundreds of thousands of people. What were the results of this trial? I think it would spoil things to let you know that at this point – all will be revealed later on.

Anyway, despite the odd hiccough on the way, by the latter half of the 20th century most people were utterly convinced that fat in the diet, saturated or otherwise, caused blood-cholesterol/LDL levels to rise. And the subsequent rise in cholesterol was overwhelmingly regarded as the primary cause of heart disease.

But it wasn't until the arrival of the statins that the cholesterol hypothesis fully conquered the world. Once it was proved that statins both lowered LDL and prevented heart disease, any remaining doubters were silenced. After all, we now had the following evidence:

- Countries with a high saturated-fat consumption have higher cholesterol levels and high deaths rates from heart disease. (See: Ancel Keys)

- People with high levels of cholesterol in the blood have high rates of heart disease. (See: Framingham Study and familial hypercholesterolaemia)

- Rationing in WWII was followed by a fall in heart-disease rates. (See: UK & Norway)

- Plaques in the arteries are full of cholesterol. (See: Virchow, Anitschkov and hundreds of other studies)

- Feed rabbits a high-cholesterol diet and they rapidly develop a high-cholesterol level and atherosclerosis. (See: Ashoff and Kritchevsky and others)

- Lowering blood cholesterol levels with statins reduces the rate of heart disease. (See: many, many clinical trials)

Sorry about bouncing around between cholesterol and LDL, but this is kind of forced on me by the fact that studies, papers and researchers keep doing the same thing. I think, though, that you get the picture. Faced with the evidence above, the case seemed open and shut. A few negative studies here and there were easily explained away. For almost everyone it was clear that the 'totality of the evidence', to use Henry Blackburn's phrase, pointed only one way. The diet-heart/cholesterol hypothesis had to be correct. Only a flat-Earth, creationist lunatic could possible argue against it.

Crikey, they must mean me. So, argue against it I shall.

CHAPTER 6

EAT WHATEVER YOU LIKE
(DIET HAS NOTHING TO DO
WITH HEART DISEASE)

At this point I am going to start dismantling the diet-heart hypothesis, starting with the question, 'Does eating a high-fat diet, or a high saturated-fat diet, cause heart disease?

I shall start by presenting all of the evidence in support of the diet-heart hypothesis. It is, as follows: [   ]. (Leave space blank for any supportive evidence that might appear.)

This time I am actually not joking. Aside from Ancel Keys's study – a study subject to accusations of selection bias – there is no evidence in support of the diet-heart hypothesis.

I believe that the strongest backing for this somewhat bold statement comes from two different sources. Firstly, the Surgeon General's office in the USA. Secondly, from Professors Law and Wald, the high priests of heart-disease orthodoxy. Both of these sources were, and remain, utterly convinced of the diet-heart hypothesis.

In 1988, the Surgeon General's office decided to gather together all the evidence linking saturated fat to heart disease, and thus silence any remaining naysayers forever. Eleven years later, the project was killed. In a letter circulated it was stated that the office *'Did not anticipate fully the magnitude of the additional expertise and staff resources that would be needed.'* After eleven years, they needed additional expertise and staff resources? What had they been doing up to then? Using a million monkeys bashing away randomly at type-writers in an attempt to produce a report?

Eleven years... Perhaps the research was hidden in a secret vault guarded by the Knights Templar, only to be discovered by de-coding centuries-old puzzles set by Leonardo da Vinci. 'Only a penitent man may enter.'

Or was it just not possible to log on to www.pubmed.org and read in about two days all the research that has ever been done. Did your Internet Service Provider have a pop-up blocker? Was that it? I know it's a fiddle to get the settings changed on your browser. But eleven years seems a long time. (Yes, I know, this was in the earliest days of the internet. But the principle remains. It isn't that difficult to track down the relevant research.)

Bill Harlan of the Oversight Committee and Associate Director of the Office of Disease Prevention at the NIH, commented: *'The report was initiated with a preconceived opinion of the conclusions, but the science behind those opinions was clearly not holding up. Clearly the thoughts of yesterday were not going to serve us very well.'*

I shall do a translation: 'We were wrong, the idea that saturated fat causes heart disease was wrong. Everything we always thought about this area is wrong. Full stop.' But no one will step that far out of line. On the surface, the world of medical research looks calm and pleasant and reasonable, like a well-tended garden with people smiling and saying things like 'with respect' and suchlike superficial pleasantries. But the world of academia is red in tooth and claw. Step out of line and you can expect no mercy. International opinion leaders guard their empires with implacable will. And crushed you will be, oh yes.

To summarise: after 11 years, the Surgeon General's office in the USA had found no evidence whatsoever to support the diet-heart hypothesis. Believe me, if they had found even the smallest scrap you would never, ever, have heard the last of it. I believe that the utter and complete failure of this organisation to support the diet-heart hypothesis represents a compelling argument against that hypothesis.

If you want more information on this particular area, go and read a paper by Gary Taubes called 'The Soft Science of Dietary Fat', published in *Science*. Several versions of his paper exist on the internet. He is good at demolishing the diet-heart hypothesis and has gathered millions of references – if you like that sort of referencing thing.

Moving on from the Surgeon General's office, it is time now to focus on Law and Wald. These two publish endless articles about the dangers of high cholesterol levels and high-fat diets and suchlike. And a few years back they proposed the concept of the Polypill. The Polypill consists of six different drugs contained within one power-packed yet 'surprisingly easy to swallow' capsule. The proposed drugs were a statin, three blood-pressure-lowering pills, aspirin and folic acid. This combination, according to the Law and Wald, should be taken by everyone, forever, to prevent heart disease. (Excuse me while I go and beat my head repeatedly against the nearest wall.)

They entitled the *BMJ* paper in which they outlined their plans 'A Strategy to Reduce Cardiovascular Disease by 80 per cent'. Pragmatically, they had patented the idea of Polypill and then published the paper in the *BMJ* setting out their arguments for it.

Anyway, Law and Wald, like the Surgeon General's office in the USA, had also noted the complete lack of evidence to support the diet-heart hypothesis. To quote directly from their teleoanalysis study, published in the *BMJ*: '*We know that saturated fat intake increases the risk of ischaemic heart disease.*' Law and Wald took the bold step of inventing a whole new scientific technique called 'teleoanalysis'.

Teleoanalysis is a technique – and I quote directly from Law and Wald – that

> ... *provides the answer to studies that would be obtained from studies that have not been done and often, for ethical and financial reasons, could never be done.*

Now, I have read this quickly. I have read it slowly. I have read it standing on my head, I have read it in my bed. But I still do not understand it. Please will someone show me the research and supporting evidence. The above quote about studies 'that have not been done' comes from Law and Wald's seminal paper 'Teleoanalysis – Combining Data from Different Types of Study'. I made several thousand copies of this paper, cut it into quarters, put a neat hole in the middle, and… I can leave the rest to your imagination.

Why did they feel the need to invent a new scientific technique? In their own words: *'A meta-analysis of randomized trials suggested that a low dietary fat intake had little effect on the risk of ischaemic heart disease.'* Translation: 'If you look at all the clinical studies that have been done, none of them has demonstrated that reducing fat in the diet has the slightest effect on heart disease.'

This, of course, had to be set beside Law and Wald's pre-existing 'knowledge'… 'that saturated fat intake increases the risk of ischaemic heart disease'. So Law and Wald looked again at the many clinical trials that had been done and came to the following conclusion: *'The effect of a significant reduction in dietary fat can easily be underestimated, even when it is based on the results of randomized trials.'*

This was their first leap forward in teleoanalytical thinking. To dismiss all the evidence from the controlled, randomised trials. How did they manage to do this? By explaining that effects can 'easily be underestimated'. How, exactly do you underestimate an effect? I fail to understand.

But this step, vital though it was, was not enough. They were left with a further problem. What evidence could they put in the place of the 'gold standard' randomised trials? They used the following:

- Firstly, the evidence that eating saturated fat raises cholesterol levels: A leads to B. [Evidence that I, for one, have not seen, but we'll let that go for the sake of this argument.]

- Secondly, the evidence that raised cholesterol levels cause heart disease: B leads to C. [See above.]

- Finally, they added the evidence that A leads to B, to the evidence that: B leads to C, and triumphantly created the evidence that A leads to C. [Thus, saturated-fat consumption does lead to heart disease.]

You think I am making this up? Well, you must read the next direct quote slowly or your brain will explode.

> *It may also be necessary to quantify the individual effects that relate to separate steps in a causal pathway – that is, the effect of factor A on disease C is determined from the estimate of the effect of A on an intermediate factor B and the estimate of the effect of B on C, rather than by directly measuring the effect of A on C. This exercise is like putting together pieces of a jigsaw puzzle.*

So there you go. In order to use the scientific technique known as teleoanalysis, you start from basics, postulate a series of experiments and estimate their likely results.

The very final stage is to combine the 'studies that could never be done' – Study Type A [otherwise known as the important and powerful studies] – to the studies that 'actually have been done' – Study Type B [otherwise known as the weak and irrelevant studies]. And, hey presto, using the following formula, you can establish that you were right all along: Study Type A + Study Type B = Study Type A. And that, ladies and gentlemen, is teleoanalysis. Don't think about it for too long, though: that way madness lies.

This is one way to keep the diet-heart hypothesis alive. Personally, I find it unbelievable that this article was written – and even more unbelievable is that it was published in the *British Medical Journal*. It is pure nonsense from start to finish.

Iam astonished that a series of estimations were used as a basis for scientific research.

Enough of Law and Wald, I banish them from my thoughts. The only thing in their paper worth remembering is the following statement: '*A meta-analysis of randomized trials suggested that a low dietary fat intake had little effect on the risk of ischaemic heart disease.'* Replace the word 'suggested' with the word 'proved', and in my opinion you are getting nearer to the truth. Add this statement to the Surgeon General's 11-year failure to establish any link between saturated fat and heart disease and you have, I believe, an answer. Even if it is a negative one.

* * * * *

Before moving on to some more directly contradictory evidence, I think it is an appropriate time to introduce two cracking quotes. The first is from Professor Michael Oliver, past president of the Royal College of Physicians in the UK. Hardly, therefore, a wild-eyed maverick loon. He wrote an article critical of the diet-heart hypothesis in *The Lancet* in 1981 and started it with the following quote from Oliver Cromwell: 'I beseech thee in the bowels of Christ, think it possible that you may be mistaken.'

But think it possible that they may be wrong, they did not, oh no.

My second quote is from Dr George Mann. He studied the Masai villagers of Kenya in the 1970s. What he found was that they had the highest cholesterol and saturated-fat intake ever discovered. Basically, they drink milk, and eat meat and fat. Yet the rate of heart disease among the Masai was virtually zero. This, along with a great deal of other evidence, led Dr George Mann, in the *New England Journal of Medicine*, to describe the diet-heart hypothesis as: 'The greatest scam in the history of medicine.'

Hear, hear.

But I'm not going to leave it there. A total lack of any supportive evidence does not necessarily prove that fat/saturated fat in the diet does not cause heart disease. Absence of evidence is not evidence of absence. Let me now mention a few of the most powerful pieces of evidence that directly contradict the diet-heart hypothesis. But where to begin? There is just so much to choose from.

I think the best place to start is with the biggest trial on dietary modification ever done, and the biggest that will ever be done – I hope.

Fifty million people were placed on a low saturated-fat diet for fourteen years. Sausages, eggs, cheese, bacon and milk were severely restricted. Fruit and fish, however, were freely available – those oh-so healthy foods.

Yes, you've guessed what I'm talking about. Rationing in the UK during and after WWII. But didn't I say that heart-disease rates fell during the war – and wasn't this used as evidence in support of the diet-heart hypothesis? Yes, I did say that. But how on earth anyone could possibly use the evidence from rationing to support the hypothesis is beyond me. Our friend teleoanalysis may be putting in an appearance again.

Fig. 19 below is a graph of heart disease rates in the UK in the years from 1928 to 1955. I know, given what I have written earlier, that perhaps it is not entirely accurate, but I don't think it is too far off. As you can see, heart disease was rising until the start of the war. There was a blip in the early years of the war, then a relentless rise. What I find particularly amusing is that the small fall in the rate of heart disease actually started in 1939, which was two years before rationing was introduced.

Fig. 19 Heart disease rates in the UK 1928–55

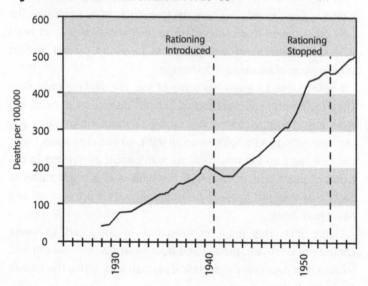

By golly, saturated fat is so deadly that even a future fall in its consumption will lead to a sudden drop in deaths from heart disease in the present! Proof that the space-time continuum is less rigid than we believe and saturated fat can leak through.

The most interesting facts to emerge about rationing are:

1: For 12 years, saturated fat consumption was severely restricted.
2: Fruit and fish consumption increased.
3: The rate of heart disease nearly trebled.

I know, it's a bit of a paradox, isn't it?

And speaking of paradoxes, I would like to introduce you to a few more. The most famous paradox is the French Paradox. The pesky French, you see, eat more saturated fat than we do in the UK. They smoke more, take less exercise, have the same cholesterol/LDL levels, the same HDL levels. They also have the same average blood pressure and the same rate of obesity. And you know what? They have one-quarter the rate of heart disease that we do. One-quarter!

In fact, the French consume more saturated fat than any other nation in Europe, and they have the lowest rate of heart disease. The only other nation that comes close to their super-low rate of heart disease is Switzerland, and the Swiss have the second highest consumption of saturated fat in Europe.

I believe that I know what some of you are thinking right now. They, the French, are protected from heart disease by drinking red wine, eating freshly cooked vegetables (all those antioxidants, you see) and eating garlic. You've read all this time and time again. I have but one word to say this. Balls! As with almost everything in the world of heart disease, people firmly believe in a whole series of 'facts' that they just know to be true, which are not true at all and never have been.

Garlic first. This magical substance is supposed to lower cholesterol levels and protect you from heart disease. You can find hundreds of papers in major clinical journals supporting this known 'fact'. For example, in 1994 a meta-analysis was published by Silagy. He looked at the effects of garlic on blood cholesterol levels, and concluded that:

> *The mean difference in reduction of total cholesterol between garlic-treated subjects and those receiving placebo (or avoiding garlic in their diet) was -0.77mmol/l. These changes represent a 12% reduction with garlic therapy beyond the final levels achieved with placebo alone.*

Pretty impressive, oui? But what were the sources for this meta-analysis?

> *A systematic review, including meta-analysis, was undertaken of published and unpublished randomized controlled trials of garlic preparation of at least four weeks duration. Studies were identified by a search of MEDLINE and the ALTERNATIVE MEDICINE electronic database from references listed and review articles, and through direct contact with garlic manufacturers.*

'... and through direct contact with garlic manufacturers'! The idea that you are willing to accept data on the effectiveness of garlic from people who make their money from manufacturing garlic capsules is an interesting one. As for the 'alternative medicine electronic databases', you might as well jump into a tent filled with hemp smoke and wait for the visions to start.

However, Silagy, to his eternal credit, went one step further. He eschewed teleoanalysis and actually did a study. A randomised, placebo-controlled study, he did. And guess what:

> *There were no significant differences between the groups receiving garlic and placebo in the mean concentrations of serum lipids, lipoproteins or Apo A1 or B, by analysis either on intention-to-treat or treatment received.*

In 1998, a group at Bonn University in Germany asked the same question. Does garlic in the diet have any impact of lipid levels in the blood? They concluded: *'We were actually surprised how clearly negative the results were.'*

Further commentary on this study came from Dr Ronald Krauss, Chairman of the American Heart Association's nutrition committee and Head of Molecular Medicine at the University of California's Lawrence Berkeley National Laboratory (another big cheese, in other words): *'This study qualifies as a solid scientific study. It's what people should be basing their thought processes on, instead of folklore.'*

So much for garlic, then. I could go on, analysing the supposed beneficial impact of red wine and lightly cooked vegetables. But if you start chasing down every single factor thought to have some impact on heart disease you will disappear up your own fundament, never to return.

Instead, I shall make a more general point. The only reason why garlic, red wine and lightly cooked vegetables were thought to protect against heart disease in the first place is the following. The French have all the major risk factors for heart disease and so they should have a rate of heart disease higher than that in the UK. But they do not. It is much, much, much lower. In order to keep the diet-heart hypothesis alive in the face of such directly contradictory evidence, a fig-leaf had to be found, and so it was. It was known that the French ate more garlic, drank more red wine and didn't cook their vegetables into a soggy tasteless mush like the ignorant Brits. Lo, as if by magic, these three factors appeared (in *The Lancet*, no less), as the explanation for the French Paradox.

But there is no evidence that any of these three factors are actually protective. NONE. By evidence, I mean a randomised, controlled clinical study. Not epidemiology, meta-analysis, discussions with French wine producers or green-leaf tea growers, or a trawl through the *Fortean Times*. In reality, the only reason that these three factors appeared was to protect the diet-heart hypothesis. They are what Karl Popper would call 'ad-hoc hypotheses', which are devices that scientists use to explain away apparent contradictions to much-loved hypotheses.

Ad-hoc hypotheses work along the following lines. You find a population with a low saturated-fat intake (and few other classical risk factors for heart disease) – yet, annoyingly, they still have a very high rate of heart disease. One such population would be Emigrant Asian Indians in the UK. The ad-hoc hypothesis used to explain away their very high rate of heart disease is, as follows. Emigrant Asian Indians are genetically predisposed to develop diabetes, which then leads to heart disease. Alakazoom! The paradox disappears.

On the other hand, if you find a population with a high saturated-fat intake, and a low rate of heart disease, e.g. the Inuit, you can always find something they do that explains why they are protected. In their case it was the high consumption of Omega 3 fatty acids from fish. Yes indeedy, this is where that particular substance first found fame, and hasn't it done well since?

This particular game has no end. In 1981, a paper was published in *Atherosclerosis* (a cracking good read), outlining 246 factors that had been identified in various studies as having an influence in heart disease. Some were protective, some causal, some were both at the same time. If this exercise were done today I can guarantee you would find well over a thousand different factors implicated in some way. Recently, just to take one example, someone suggested that the much lower rate of heart disease in south-west France, compared to north-east France, was because the saturated fat they ate was different. In the south-west they ate more pork fat and less beef fat. So now it is no longer simply saturated fat that is deadly, it is the precise type of saturated fat, in precise proportions. Just how finely can one hypothesis be sliced before it becomes thin air?

What this highlights, to me at least, is one simple fact. Once someone decided that saturated fat causes heart disease, then NOTHING will change their minds. There is no evidence that cannot be dismissed in one way or another. And there is also no end to the development of new ad-hoc hypotheses. You can just keep plucking them out of the air endlessly – no proof required.

Genetic predisposition is one of the most commonly used 'explain-all' ad-hoc hypotheses, and it is a particular bug-bear of mine. Someone

I knew quite well had a heart attack recently, aged 36. He was very fit, almost to international level at cycling. He was also extremely thin. His resting pulse was 50 a minute, his blood pressure was 120/70 (bang on normal). His total cholesterol level was 3.0mmol/l, which is very low. He was vegetarian and a non-smoker. I know what you're thinking: he deserved it. Steady, he's a nice bloke, actually, if a bit worthy.

Now, you can go through all the risk factors tables produced by the American Heart Association, the European Society of Cardiology and the British Heart Foundation – and any other cardiology society you care to mention. According to the lot of them, he had no risk factors. Therefore, he should not have had a heart attack. However, it did emerge that his father had a heart attack aged 50. A-ha! He was genetically susceptible, then! Phew, there's your answer. I beg to differ: if you think about this in any depth, it is a completely idiotic statement to make.

If someone is genetically susceptible to heart disease, that susceptibility must operate though some identifiable mechanism. Or does a big finger suddenly appear from the sky and go: 'Pow! Heart attack time, bad luck.' Genetically susceptible people don't need high LDL levels, or high blood pressure. They don't need to smoke or eat a high-fat diet. They don't need to be overweight, or have diabetes – or anything, actually. They are felled by a mysterious genetic force, operating in a way that no one can detect.

Other people are killed by risk factors. But such factors count for nothing if you are genetically susceptible. I have one word to say to this – and it's a word I've used before in a similar context. Balls.

Karl Popper recognised such reasoning. He called it the use of circular logic. His example, was as follows:

Consider the following dialogue: 'Why is the sea so rough today?' – 'Because Neptune is very angry' – 'By what evidence can you support your statement that Neptune is very angry?' – 'Oh, don't you see how very rough the sea is? And is it not always rough when Neptune is angry?'

Popper, K. Popper Selections

I would ask you to consider the following dialogue:

> 'Why has this man, with no risk factors for heart disease, had a heart attack?' – 'Because he is genetically susceptible.' – 'By what evidence can you support your statement that he is genetically susceptible?' 'Oh, don't you see that he has had a heart attack, although he has no risk factors? So he must be genetically susceptible.'

If you are going to suggest that people are genetically susceptible to heart disease, then you also have to attempt to explain the mechanism. Otherwise, you might as well believe in magic. 'Abracadabra, genetics – heart attack.' Alternatively, you could accept that the mainstream risk factors are not, actually, risk factors at all – since you can have a heart attack without having any of them. Your choice.

As ever, I have drifted off track a bit. But I wanted to highlight the endless games that people play to keep the diet-heart hypothesis alive. There is always a reason why population X and their paradoxical rate of heart disease does not mean that the diet-heart hypothesis is wrong. And once you have 246 factors to throw into the mix, you can complicate matters by a zillion: 'Oh, you didn't measure this, or that…' Then, if all else fails, you can just throw in the dreaded word 'multifactorial'. End of discussion. End of will to live.

However, despite the fact that any paradox discovered is immediately 'ad-hocced' into non-existence, I thought I would introduce you to a couple more paradoxes before leaving this discussion. Firstly, the Israeli Paradox.

> *Israel has one of the highest dietary polyunsaturated/saturated fat ratios in the world; the consumption of Omega-6 polyunsaturated fatty acids (PUFA) is about 8% higher than in the USA, and 10–12% higher than in most European countries. In fact, Israeli Jews may be regarded as a population-based dietary experiment of the effect of a high Omega-6 PUFA diet… Despite such national habits, there is paradoxically a high prevalence of*

cardiovascular diseases, hypertension, non-insulin-dependent diabetes mellitus and obesity.[6]

I will allow you to guess what the response to this finding was. Go on, you know you can do it. The response was to suggest that Omega 6 polyunsaturated fats are dangerous, at least they are if the proportion of Omega 6 to Omega 3 exceeds a ratio of 4:1... or perhaps it was if Jupiter is out of alignment with Venus in the sign of Libra.

Here's another paradox. After WWII, saturated-fat consumption in Switzerland increased by 20 per cent. Yet during this 25-year period, the rate of heart disease fell. It is now clearly established, of course, that Swiss cows produce cheese high in Omega 3 fatty acids.

> *The researchers observed a trend. Cheeses from the milk of purely grass-fed alpine cows had the best fat profile, followed by cheeses from silage-fed alpine cows and linseed-supplemented cows. Lowest in Omega 3 fatty acids were the Emmentalers and then the Cheddars. Grass-based alpine cheese contained four times as much of the plant Omega-3 ALA as did the Cheddar, more Omega 3 fats in general, three times as much conjugated linoleic acid, and 20 percent less of the saturated fat palmitic acid.*
>
> *http://www.sciencenews.org/articles/20040124/food.asp*

This passage has the advantage of being completely incomprehensible to all but the most dedicated follower of fat biochemistry. However, it clearly suggests something about Omega 3 fatty acids being at higher levels in alpine-fed cows. 'A-ha... so that's' why the Swiss rate of heart disease fell,' he exclaimed, before his brain finally turned to mush.

I could go on and on. But I hope you get the general drift that there is actually no end, ever, to the ability of researchers to come up with a

---

6: Yam, D. Eliraz, A. Berry, EM. 'Diet and Disease – the Israeli Paradox: Possible Dangers of a high Omega-6 Polyunsaturated Fatty Acid Diet'. Isr J Med Sci, November 1996; 32(11): 1134–43.

reason why every single paradox is not really a paradox at all. And why a high saturated-fat diet really does cause heart disease. I would just ask, how many paradoxes do you need before the only paradox left is the diet-heart hypothesis itself?

Of course, it you wish to believe all of the ad-hoc hypotheses currently in existence, it seems that you are allowed to eat saturated fat and remain healthy. But only if you eat saturated pork fat, and cheese from cows eating grass in a high alpine pasture in Switzerland, but make sure it is cheddar and not Emmental – or was that the other way round?

Golly, it sure is tricky eating a healthy diet. You need a biochemist on hand, equipped with a mass spectrometer and a three-dimensional crystallography x-ray machine, lest an unhealthy fat were to slip through. 'Hold on, that's an unconjugated linoleic acid molecule, don't move, don't swallow... I think I can just reach it...'

Before I finish let's just run through a couple of the more spectacular studies contradicting the idea that saturated fat causes heart disease. I will then present you with two graphs that might finally persuade you that a diet high in saturated fat has nothing to with heart disease.

1: MALMO: SWEDEN (2005)[8]

- 28,098 middle-aged men and women
- Split into four categories (quartiles) from low to high fat/saturated-fat intake
- Follow-up: 6.6 years

Findings

Saturated fat showed no relationship with cardiovascular disease in men. Among women, cardiovascular mortality showed a downward trend with increasing saturated-fat intake, but the relative risk reductions did not reach statistical significance. (In other words, there was no difference.)

8 Leosdottir, M. Nilsson, PM. Nilsson, JA. Mansson, H. Berglund, G. 'Dietary fat intake and early mortality patterns – data from The Malmo Diet and Cancer Study'. J Intern Med, August 2005; 258(2): 153–65.

Conclusions

'With our results added to the pool of evidence from large-scale prospective cohort studies on dietary fat, disease and mortality, traditional dietary guidelines concerning fat intake are thus generally not strongly supported.'

As ever, the conclusion is vague and somewhat apologetic: '... traditional dietary guidelines concerning fat intake are thus generally not strongly supported.' Come on, chaps, show a bit of a stiff upper lip! According to this study, the traditional dietary guidelines are utter bunk. Shout it loudly from the hilltops! Climb every mountain, ford every stream! Shoot every Omega 3 cow!

2: WOMEN'S HEALTH INTERVENTION USA (2006)

- 48,835 women aged 50 to 79
- Study length: 8.1 years
- Major intervention in diet (i.e., this was not a passive observational trial. This was a randomised, interventional, controlled clinical study involving almost fifty thousand women. The gold standard.)

Those randomised to the intervention group were intensively counselled to reduce their daily fat intake to twenty per cent of calories, to increase their intake of fruits and vegetables to at least five servings daily, and to increase grain consumption to at least six servings daily. By the sixth year, the intervention group was consuming, on average, 29 per cent of calories as fat, compared to 37 per cent in the control group. The corresponding figures for saturated fat were 9.5 per cent and 12.4 per cent, respectively.

Findings

Among the study population as a whole, there were no significant differences in CHD or stroke incidence, CHD or stroke mortality, or total mortality. And, in addition, the low-fat diet produced no reduction in the incidence or mortality rates of breast cancer, colorectal cancer, or total cancer either.

I thought you might find it interesting to read the 'establishment' interpretation of this trial:

> *'The results of this study do not change established recommen-dations on disease prevention. Women should continue to get regular mammograms and screenings for colorectal cancer, and work with their doctors to reduce their risks for heart disease including following a diet low in saturated fat, trans fat and cholesterol,' said National Heart, Lung, and Blood Institute Director Elizabeth G Nabel, MD.*
>
> (I would have concluded the exact
> opposite from the same study!)

> *'This study shows that just reducing total fat intake does not go far enough to have an impact on heart disease risk. While the participants' overall change in LDL "bad" cholesterol was small, we saw trends towards greater reductions in cholesterol and heart disease risk in women eating less saturated and trans fat,' said Jacques Rossouw, MD, WHI project officer.*
>
> ('We saw trends'. I must have missed something.)

> *Judy O'Sullivan, a cardiac nurse at the British Heart Foundation, said: 'Numerous studies have confirmed there are huge heart benefits from maintaining a healthy lifestyle which involves a balanced diet and regular physical activity. It is easy to identify a number of important reasons why this study did not agree with previous research.'*
>
> (Go on then, Judy, identify them.)

(Now for my favourite quote):'There may have been some "disappoint-ment" that the studies didn't always give clear answers,' acknowledges Dr Elizabeth Nabel, heart chief at the National Institutes of Health.'The findings are what they are… Now we're in a second wave of putting the findings into perspective.'

'Putting the findings into perspective.' Perhaps the findings merely represent a 'paradox'; if not, I am sure that plenty of ad-hoc hypotheses will emerge which will sweep this $400-million-dollar trial into the dustbin.

DR KENDRICK'S 14-COUNTRY STUDY

I shall now give you twice as much research for your money as Ancel Keys. I looked at the figures gathered by the World Health Organization on saturated-fat consumption and heart-disease rates in various countries throughout Europe. All figures are from 1998, or within two years of 1998 if figures for that exact year were not available.

I looked first at the seven countries with the lowest consumption of saturated fat, and compared this to their rate of heart disease. I then took the seven countries with the highest consumption of saturated fat and compared this to their rate of heart disease (see Figs 18 and 19, below and opposite):

Fig 18 Comparison of heart disease deaths vs consumption of saturated fat % calories

(Countries with lowest saturated-fat consumption)

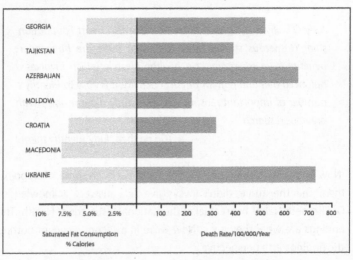

Fig 19 Comparison of heart disease deaths vs consumption of saturated fat % calories

(Countries with highest saturated-fat consumption)

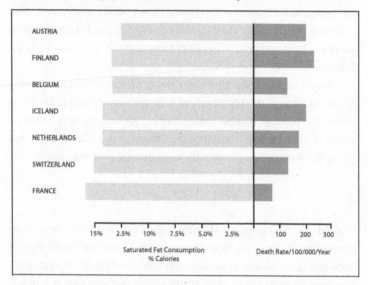

AUSTRIA
FINLAND
BELGIUM
ICELAND
NETHERLANDS
SWITZERLAND
FRANCE

15%   2.5%   10%   7.5%   5.0%   2.5%   100   200   300

Saturated Fat Consumption   Death Rate/100/000/Year
% Calories

When I first showed these graphs to another doctor he exclaimed: 'My goodness, saturated fat is worse for you than I thought!' To me, this just goes to show that, even when confronted with the facts, people still view them through preconceived prejudices.

I then took him through the graphs more slowly, pointing out that he had got it completely the wrong way round. The facts are:

- Every single one of the seven countries with the lowest saturated-fat consumption has significantly higher rates of heart disease than every single one of the seven countries with the highest saturated-fat consumption.

At which point his immediate response was: 'This can't be right, where did you get this rubbish from?'

I then showed him the original figures, pointing out that they came from the World Health Organization. He then said, 'Well there obviously must be other factors involved.' What he would not do, however, was accept that there is no connection between saturated fat consumption and heart disease. Even when confronted with evidence that is, in my view, overwhelming. Far more overwhelming, ironically, than anything Ancel Keys managed to come up with in the first place.

Now, of course, I know that there has to be some reason why every single country in the top seven of saturated fat consumption has a lower rate of heart disease than every single country in the bottom seven of saturated-fat consumption. Whatever it is, though, it is not going to have anything to do with saturated-fat consumption.

* * * * *

I could fill an entire book with studies that have been done contradicting the diet-heart hypothesis. There are even studies showing, quite clearly, that reducing saturated fat is harmful. But I feel that quoting study after study would get somewhat tedious. However, if you are interested in looking into this area in more detail, there are several very good and well-written sources of information where you can read about such trials to your heart's content. Here are three of them:

www.thincs.org
www.theomnivore.com
www.second-opinions.co.uk

Just before signing off on this chapter, I need to make an admission. Despite my slagging off all ad-hoc hypotheses, and their feeble use as crutches to support the diet-heart hypothesis, two dietary substances appear to have surfaced that do seem to be consistently beneficial in protecting against heart disease.

1: Omega 3 fatty acids.

This type of fat appears to have two effects that may be protective. Firstly, it has a reasonably strong anti-coagulant effect, a bit like aspirin. Secondly, it seems to protect against heart arrhythmias. (Omega 3 fatty acids, it should be added, have no effect on LDL levels.) You tend to find Omega 3-type fats in fish. So, although it rather sticks in my craw, I feel I must recommend that Omega 3 fats are probably good for you.

2: Alcohol

Moderate alcohol consumption does appear to reduce the risk of dying of heart disease by about twenty per cent, on average. The type of alcohol is more or less irrelevant (although wine and beer seem better than spirits). However, extremely heavy or binge drinking seems to have the opposite effect. This may be due to the fact that after a very heavy drinking session, the blood-clotting system can 'rebound', making blood clots more likely to form.

POSTSCRIPT

A few of my favourite quotes

It had been noted in the Framingham Study that a high saturated fat consumption reduced the rate of strokes. It was suggested that, because strokes tend to affect older men, the fatty diet was causing those in the trial to die of heart disease before they could die of a stroke (yes, it's yet another desperate ad-hoc hypothesis). But the researchers discounted this, saying:

> This hypothesis, however, depends on the presence of a strong direct association of fat intake with coronary heart disease. Since we found no such association, competing mortality from coronary heart disease is very unlikely to explain our results.

It had to be dragged out of them. But after 49 years, which is a pretty long time period for any study, the Framingham Study flatly contradicts the diet-heart hypothesis.

The overall results do not show a beneficial effect on coronary heart disease or total mortality from this multifactor intervention.

The above quote is from the Multiple Risk Factor Intervention Trial (MR-FIT) involving 28 medical centres, 250 researchers and 361,662 men. Cholesterol consumption was cut by 42 per cent, saturated fat consumption by 28 per cent. With no effect on heart disease.

As multiple intervention against risk factors for coronary heart disease in middle-aged men at only moderate risk seem to have failed to reduce both morbidity and mortality such interventions become increasingly difficult to justify. This runs counter to the recommendations of many national and international advisory bodies which must now take the recent findings from Finland into consideration. Not to do so may be ethically unacceptable.

This is a quote from Professor Michael Oliver, and follows a study in Finland. In a ten-year follow-up to the initial study (hailed as a success) it found that those people who continued to follow the carefully controlled cholesterol-lowering diet were twice as likely to die of heart disease as those who didn't.

Final word goes to American cardiologist EH Ahrens, Jr. Initially a supporter of the low-fat diet, after 25 years of research he concluded that:

If the public's diet is going to be decided by popularity polls and with diminishing regard for the scientific evidence, I fear that future generations will be left in ignorance of the real merits, as well as the possible faults in any dietary regimen aimed at prevention of coronary heart disease.

He is much more polite than I.

CHAPTER 7

A RAISED CHOLESTEROL/LDL LEVEL DOES NOT CAUSE HEART DISEASE

At this point in the book, I move off the edge of the charts and into unexplored lands marked 'Here be dragons.' For while it's true that the bulk of the mainstream still supports the diet part of the diet-heart hypothesis, there are many researchers who have long since given up on the idea – including such notables as Professor Michael Oliver. So I am far from being a lonely traveller in that area.

But when it comes to attacking the second part of the hypothesis, namely that raised cholesterol levels cause heart disease, I find myself in the wilderness. There are a few others moving around in this landscape, true, but not many. To be frank, a number of them have a tendency to write in green ink and regularly howl at the moon, whereas I only howl at a full moon.

I am also fully aware that when I talk about raised cholesterol levels causing heart disease I am in the realm of the 'known fact' – a fact that has apparently been proven beyond the slightest doubt, time and time again.

However, despite that fact that hardly anyone else agrees with me, I believe firmly that the cholesterol hypothesis is wrong. By the time you have finished this chapter, I hope to have convinced you of this fact too.

Before starting on the demolition job I must admit that, for many years, I too believed that a raised cholesterol level caused heart disease.

On the face of it the evidence seemed overwhelming, and it also seemed to make sense. The most powerful facts, at least to me, were the following:

Fact One: Atherosclerotic plaques contain a lot of cholesterol, which must have come from the blood. So heart disease had to have something to do with cholesterol-containing lipoproteins.

Fact Two: People with familial hypercholesterolaemia (FH) die very young from heart disease, sometimes as young as five.

Fact Three: Statins lower cholesterol levels and protect against heart disease.

Fact Four: 'Normal' people (without FH) with higher cholesterol levels are more likely to die from heart disease.

These facts seemed concrete and inarguable. Every time I opened a journal, or read a paper, they were confirmed. Again and again.

But these facts are really only partially true. They are rather like the false-fronted buildings used in Westerns. If you look at them from dead ahead, you see what looks like an entire town laid out in front of you. But if you move sideways, just a little bit, you can see that the supposedly solid buildings are just four-inch-thick plywood with nothing behind them at all.

And so it is with the second part of the cholesterol hypothesis – 'raised cholesterol/LDL causes CHD'. Seen from one angle, the facts look solid. But once you decide to quit the 'opinion leader guided tour', you get a completely different view. And so, ladies and gentlemen, it is time for a backstage trip around the cholesterol hypothesis.

Gasp as you see the real facts exposed for the first time!

Scream as the fearsome Austrian study bares it claws! Prepare to be amazed as the awesome three-headed Honolulu trial eats LDL in front of your very eyes!

Roll up, roll up. Only two and thruppence for adults, and children under six are free!

CHOLESTEROL LEVELS AND STROKES

I shall start the discussion by moving sideways for a moment to talk about a slightly different manifestation of cardiovascular disease – strokes. Why am I talking about strokes instead of heart disease? Well, strokes and heart disease are part of the family known as cardiovascular disease (CVD). People with heart disease are far more likely to get strokes, and vice versa. Strokes also kill very nearly as many people as heart attacks, so this is not some minor problem.

A stroke happens when blood supply to a part of the brain is cut off. The brain tissue downstream dies, and the victim will lose some brain function. A small stroke is sometimes known as a transient ischaemic attack (TIA); a big stroke can be fatal, or leave the victim with severe disability.

The most common cause of a stroke is the development of a big, nasty atherosclerotic plaque at the base of neck, in the carotid arteries. Clots form over these plaques. The clots can then break off and travel into the brain, where they get jammed into an artery and block the blood flow.

Given the fact that both strokes and heart disease are caused by the development of atherosclerotic plaques, you would think, would you not, that if a raised cholesterol level is a risk factor for heart disease, it would also be a risk factor for stroke? But it is not.

In 1995, *The Lancet* published a massive study that looked at 450,000 people over a period of 16 years who suffered, between them, 13,000 strokes. This represented 7.3 million person-years of observation. Frankly, that's quite long enough for anybody. And the conclusions thereof: *'There was no association between blood cholesterol and stroke.'*

More recently, a pan-European study known as EUROSTROKE, published in 2002, asked the same question. The result: *'This analysis of the EUROSTROKE project could not disclose an association of total cholesterol with fatal, non-fatal, haemorrhagic or ischaemic stroke.'*

There are many other studies showing exactly the same thing. So, you have two conditions – stroke and heart disease – that are both fundamentally a form of arterial disease. Yet, raised cholesterol is a risk factor for one, but not the other. Listed below is a slightly shortened list of risk factors for stroke from the American Stroke Association:

- High blood pressure
- Tobacco use
- Diabetes
- Carotid or other artery disease
- Other heart disease – people with coronary heart disease or heart failure have a higher risk of stroke
- Physical inactivity and obesity
- Excessive alcohol intake
- Some illegal drugs – intravenous drug abuse carries a high risk of stroke
- Cocaine use has been linked to strokes and heart attacks
- Increasing age
- Sex (gender) – stroke is more common in men than in women
- Prior stroke or heart attack – someone who has had a stroke is at much higher risk of having another one. If you've had a heart attack, you're at higher risk of having a stroke too

Given that these are precisely the same risk factors as for heart disease (in fact, some of them are heart disease), where is cholesterol in this list? Even more critical for this discussion, how can lowering cholesterol with statins reduce the risk of stroke (which they do), if a raised cholesterol level isn't a risk factor for stroke? This most certainly does not make sense.

Actually, it would make perfect sense if you believe that any benefit gained from taking a statin has nothing to do with lowering cholesterol levels. But this explanation cannot be allowed by the medicine world at large, or else the entire cholesterol hypothesis crumbles to the ground.

In fact, in its quiet, academic sort of way, this was a crisis! The inner keep of the castle was under fire, the enemy had got in unnoticed through an underground tunnel. No one had expected an attack from this direction. The cholesterol hypothesis had to be protected. But how? How indeed. Tricky, this one. Very tricky.

But you know, the cholesterol brotherhood has some very clever boffins on its side. Although, in this area I think we should trust the instincts of Montaigne:

> *I prefer the company of peasants because they have not been educated sufficiently to reason incorrectly.*
>
> *Michel de Montaigne*

By the way,

> *I quote others only in order the better to express myself.*
>
> *Michel de Montaigne*

Step one to protect the cholesterol hypothesis was to split strokes into two basic types.

- Ischaemic
- Haemorrhagic

An ischaemic stroke is caused when a small blood clot travels into the brain, then gets jammed as the arteries narrow. The bigger the clot, the bigger the artery that gets blocked and the bigger the stroke. Around 75 per cent of strokes are ischaemic.

A haemorrhagic stroke happens when an artery in the brain

bursts. This causes blood to escape into the brain tissue and cause damage. Haemorrhagic strokes are, generally, more deadly than ischaemic strokes.

Once you have split strokes into two types, you then state that an increased cholesterol level causes ischaemic strokes. On the other hand, a low cholesterol level does not cause haemorrhagic strokes, it is merely associated with haemorrhagic strokes. (Yet another ad-hoc hypothesis plucked from thin air.)

Then – goodness me, this is getting complicated – if you lower cholesterol levels, you will prevent ischaemic strokes, but you will not cause an increase in haemorrhagic strokes. Which is why lowering cholesterol levels with statins can reduce the overall rate of stroke – even if a raised cholesterol level is not a risk factor for stroke. Phew! I'm glad we sorted that one out.

At which point you can add in the one missing risk factor from the American Stroke Association list. Yes, it's cholesterol. I cut it out of the list – what a naughty boy. But I did it for a reason. Now you can read it with open eyes:

> *A high level of total cholesterol in the blood (240 mg/dL or higher [about 6 mmol/l]) is a major risk factor for heart disease, which raises your risk of stroke. Recent studies show that high levels of LDL ['bad'] cholesterol (greater than 100 mg/dL [about 3 mmol/l]) and triglycerides (blood fats, 150 mg/dL or higher [about 4.5 mmol/l]) increase the risk of stroke in people with previous coronary heart disease, ischemic stroke or transient ischemic attack (TIA).*
>
> *http://www.americanheart.org/presenter.jhtml?identifier=4716*

This is so carefully crafted that if you read it without prior knowledge you would think it said that increased cholesterol levels increase the risk of stroke. But it doesn't. What it says – if you read it very carefully – is that a high cholesterol level is a major risk for heart disease – and heart disease, in turn, increases your risk of stroke. Hmmmm! This is teleoanalysis again:

- A (a raised cholesterol level) leads to B (heart disease).
- B (heart disease) causes C (stroke).
- A isn't a risk factor for C in any study.
- But A acting through B causes C.
- Thus, A does cause C – huzzah! Faultless logic.

The American Stroke Association then goes on to state that raised LDL levels increase the risk of stroke – in people who already have heart disease, or who have already suffered a stroke. Now, I could chase myself round in circles trying to dissect the logic in that passage. But I will just make one point. What this passage does not say is that raised cholesterol is a risk factor for stroke. Why not? Because that would be a lie. And the powers that be do not lie – they just ensure that the truth lies sleeping atop a very high tower, guarded by fierce beasties with awfully sharp teeth.

As a general point, I will just say that it is a damn sight easier to create ad-hoc hypotheses, and pluck conjectures from the sky, than it is to disprove them. Usually, by the time you have managed to do so, everyone's eyes have glazed over. Or the whole argument has become so complex that you forget where you started.

But I am going to hunt this one down, because I believe it is kind of critical. What I am going to show you is that a low cholesterol level is actually associated with a massive increase in death from stroke, and may even be a cause. Let's start with a helpful little passage:

> Epidemiological data are generally consistent with the animal experiments, they indicate that diets which are very low in fat increase the occurrence of some forms of stroke. Societies with a low intake of fat and animal protein, such as traditional Japan, tend to have high rates of haemorrhagic stroke. An elevated risk of stroke is found among segments of the Japanese population with low levels of serum cholesterol, particularly among those with high blood pressure.
>
> In a large, screened population of men in the USA, those with

the lowest serum cholesterol levels had an elevated risk of haemorrhagic stroke.

http://www.fao.org/docrep/V4700E/V4700E0i.htm

This suggests that a low cholesterol level may actually cause haemorrhagic stroke. Is this effect powerful enough overcome the theoretical benefits of low cholesterol in preventing ischaemic stroke? To answer this question, we need to move to Japan, land of the rising sun and the falling stroke. While the Japanese have always had a low rate of heart disease, they used to have the highest rate of strokes in the world. At one time their rate of stroke was 30 times their rate of heart attacks.

In fact, death from stroke represented such a huge health problem that, in the not-too-distant past, the Japanese were being actively encouraged to raise their fat intake to prevent so many of them dying of strokes. This was probably good advice, as confirmed by a 15-year Japanese study published in *Stroke* in 2004:

> *The risk of death from [cerebral] infarction [AKA stroke] was reduced by 64% in the high cholesterol consumption group, compared with the low cholesterol consumption group... Animal protein was not significantly associated with [cerebral] infarction after adjustment for animal fat and cholesterol...*
>
> *This study suggests that in Japan, where animal product intake is lower than in Western countries, a high consumption of animal fat and cholesterol was associated with a reduced risk of cerebral infarction death.*

Compare and contrast this hugely positive result with the miserable failure in any trial to show that reducing saturated fat in the diet prevents heart disease. I know that I am supposed to have moved on from discussing the diet-heart hypothesis, but hey! This is just too good to resist! A high consumption of saturated fat reduces the stroke rate by 64 per cent. Reducing saturated fat in the diet reduces the risk of heart disease by 0 per cent.

Perhaps as a result of the advice to increase fat consumption, or perhaps as a result of enemy infiltration by fast food restaurants, in the last 50 years fat, and saturated fat, consumption has gone up in Japan, as have cholesterol levels. (See table below.)

Changes in Japanese diet, 1958–99

	1958	1999
Total Calories	2,837	2,202
Carbohydrate intake % calories	84	62
Protein intake % calories	11	18
Fat intake % calories	5	20

Virtually a doubling of protein intake, and a quadrupling of fat intake. Oh my God, what happened to the cholesterol levels? They went up by 20 per cent:

Cholesterol levels 1958 = 3.9mmol/l
Cholesterol levels 1999 = 4.9mmol/l

The poor devils, they must have started to drop like flies from heart disease. Ah, no.

Fig. 20 CHD mortality in Japanese men, 1965–95

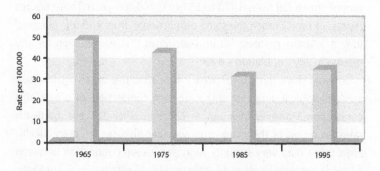

And just look what has happened to the rate of stroke:

Fig. 21 Death rates from stroke in Japanese men (aged 60–69), 1950–95

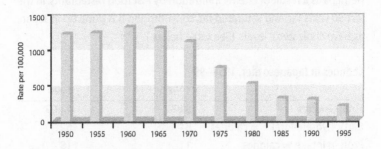

Good golly, Miss Molly! I think we have another paradox on our hands. A double paradox, no less. If a raised cholesterol level does actually cause ischaemic stroke, and 75 per cent of strokes are ischaemic, then a 20 per cent rise in cholesterol levels across the board ought to – really ought to – increase the rate of stroke. (Note: this graph does not distinguish between the two types of stroke.) Instead, between 1965 and 1995 the rate of stroke fell from 1,334 to 226 (per 100,000/year). This is a 5.9-fold reduction. Five point nine. You know, that's very nearly six.

And if you are wondering why I chose the age group 60–69, it wasn't because this particular age make my case stronger. It just seemed a reasonable age to look at. Had I chosen men aged 55–59, the rate of stroke fell from 463 to 81 (per 100,000/year). If I had chosen 75–79, the rate of stroke fell from 3,470 to 851 (per 100,000/year). These figures represent pretty much the same proportional drop. And it is gigantic. In fact, it is the greatest fall in death rates I have ever seen for any disease in any population – ever.

So what does this prove? Well, it doesn't prove anything, because epidemiological data can only suggest a connection, or a lack of a connection. However, in Japan, as cholesterol levels went up, death rates from two of the main cardiovascular diseases fell dramatically. Ergo, these data very strongly suggest a causal connection between raised cholesterol levels and cardiovascular disease is [   ] unlikely. (Insert adverb of your choice into the brackets above.)

You can splutter all you like about paradoxes, and that one country 'does not prove anything'. Japan may be just one country, but it is a country of 115 million people. So, in reality, it is 115 million inscrutable paradoxes. I think if I did a clinical trial on 115 million people, most scientists would consider that to be adequately 'powered' to disprove the null hypothesis (don't worry, just a bit of statistical jargon).

My takeaway point in this section on strokes is as follows. According to mainstream thinking, ischaemic strokes are caused by raised cholesterol levels, and ischaemic strokes represent 75 per cent of all strokes. However, over the last 50 years, cholesterol levels have risen by 20 per cent in Japan, and the rate of stroke has fallen off the edge of a cliff – dropping 600 per cent. And the rate of heart disease has also fallen dramatically. Gentlemen, try to fit those pieces of a jigsaw puzzle together. (Here's a hint. Some of the pieces may, currently, be upside down.)

CHOLESTEROL/LDL AND TOTAL MORTALITY

Having looked at stroke, and the evidence that the greatest risk factor for stroke is a low cholesterol level, not a high cholesterol level, I think that it is time to introduce the concept of 'total mortality'.

You see, it is actually possible to die of things other than heart disease, although to hear a cardiologist speak you would sometimes think not. They are utterly obsessed with cardiovascular deaths. Benefits in this area are trumpeted to the very skies. Yet overall mortality is often overlooked; in some trials these data isn't even published at all.

Speaking personally, I think that total mortality data are by far the most important thing. I'm not that bothered about exactly how people die. Nor, I suspect, are most people. It's the dying bit we are all trying to prevent, or avoid. Indeed, to be perfectly honest, a massive heart attack seems preferable to dying slowly of cancer. Maybe you think not. It's probably a matter of personal taste. So I think it is interesting to look rather more closely at the association between cholesterol levels and total mortality. That is, mortality from everything. Heart disease, cancer, respiratory diseases, digestive diseases – the works.

Time, then, to look at the Conference on Low Blood Cholesterol and Mortality, which gathered together the data from 523,737 men and 124,814 women, and reported back in 1992. I think you should probably go and make yourself a cup of coffee at this point, because I do not think you are going to believe the data that I am about to present. So steady yourself.

Firstly, the overall mortality data from women:

Fig. 22 Risk of death at various cholesterol levels in the next five years – women

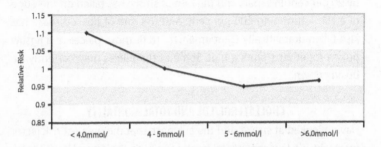

I think that's pretty clear, it is not? The healthiest cholesterol level is somewhere around about 5.5mmol/l. I know that this data is on total cholesterol, not LDL. But I can assure you that the two things are tightly bound. In study after study, total cholesterol was as good a predictor of death as LDL alone – if not better. And a higher total cholesterol level means, 99 per cent of the time, a higher LDL level.

Now, someone like me might look at that data and wonder why the current recommendations are that we should all strive to get the cholesterol level below 5.0mmol/l. Indeed, the most recent guidelines recommend that we should be aiming to get below 4.0mmol/l. To be frank, one look at the diagram on female mortality should tell you everything you need to know about that idea. (Top tip: look to the left and upwards on the graph.)

Anyway, on to men and total mortality:

Fig.23 Risk of death at various cholesterol levels in the next five years – men

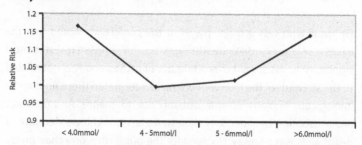

Not quite the same pattern as with women, more of a U-shaped curve. But it's still hardly a graph that suggests cholesterol is a deadly killer, as the highest mortality rate is to be found at the lowest cholesterol level.

Just for the heck of it, below is a graph showing the rate of non-cancer, non-cardiovascular mortality in women. This one just keeps going down as cholesterol levels go up:

Fig. 24 Risk of non-cancer non-cardiovascular death at various cholesterol levels in the next five years – women

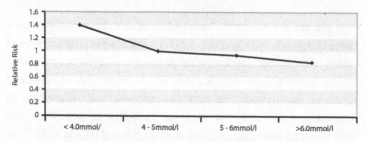

But you shouldn't worry about low cholesterol levels. Why not? Because no one at the conference did:

> *Most participants considered it to be likely that many of the statistical associations of low or lowered TC (total cholesterol) level are explainable by confounding in one form or another. The conference focused on the apparent existence and nature of these*

*associations and on the need to understand their source, rather
than on any pertinence of the finding for public health policy.*

Dr Yusuf, who was a major player at the conference, noted that the excess of non-cardiac deaths was: '... of borderline statistical significance, was spread over a number of causes, and was not related to the strength of the intervention'. Yusuf interpreted these findings as 'biologically implausible and probably due to chance'. And thus was any association between low cholesterol levels and increased rate of death airily waved away. No need for the public to worry their pretty little heads about such matters.

But you know, perhaps the public should worry their pretty little heads. Because a key finding from the Framingham Study was the following.

*There is a direct association between falling cholesterol levels over
the first 14 years [of the study] and mortality over the following 18
years (11% overall and 14% CVD death rate increase per 1mg/dl
per year drop in cholesterol levels).*

Yes, you did just read that. Those people whose cholesterol levels fell, were at a greatly increased risk of dying – and at an even greater risk of dying of cardiovascular disease. I shall expand on these figures a bit.

The figures on total mortality show an 11 per cent overall increase of death for each 1mg/dl drop in cholesterol levels, which doesn't sound that bad. But remember that mg/dl are titchy little US units. To convert into the magnificent jumbo-sized units used in the UK – mmol/l – you need to multiply by 39. So, a quick translation of the Framingham results gives the following: a 1mmol/l fall in cholesterol levels is equal to a (39 x 11 per cent) increase in the risk of total mortality. Which is 429 per cent.

To put this into a real-life context, if your total cholesterol were to fall from 5 to 4 mmol/l, your risk of dying would increase by more than 400 per cent. Not only that, but your risk of dying of a cardiovascular disease would increase by 39 x 14 per cent = 546 per cent.

This might seem so incredible that you may not believe that you read it. But I can assure you that it is there, in black and white, in the *Journal of the American Medical Association*, 24 April 1987, pages 2176 to 2180: 'Cholesterol and mortality. 30 years of follow-up from the Framingham Study'.

I hope you recognise by now that I make up nothing. All facts and data that I use come from peer-reviewed, high-impact journals that can be found by looking in the database, www.pubmed.org – a fantastic resource that is absolutely free.

The interpretation of those facts, however – that's a completely different matter. A few statistical models here, a bit of meta-analysis there, just a sprinkling of confounding variables, a few 'probably due to chances' thrown into the mix and, bibbity, bobbity, boo! A circle turns into a square, and cholesterol turns into a deadly killer.

But it is time to return the main point of this particular story, which is that a low cholesterol level, especially after the age of 50, significantly increases your risk of dying. One massive long-lasting study that looked specifically at cholesterol levels and mortality in older people, was carried out in Honolulu and published in August 2001 in *The Lancet*. And the findings thereof:

> *Our data accord with previous findings of increased mortality in elderly people with low serum cholesterol, and show that long term persistence of low cholesterol concentration actually increases the risk of death. Thus, the earlier that patients start to have lower cholesterol concentrations, the greater the risk of death.*

Their interpretation:

> *We have been unable to explain our results. These data cast doubt on the scientific justification for lowering cholesterol to very low concentrations.*

This study, by the way, was immediately attacked from all sides. I think my favourite attack included the word 'irresponsible'. Things have come to a pretty pass when publishing a well-designed medical study in *The Lancet* is considered irresponsible. I mean, people might learn the truth and then there is no way of knowing what will happen. Panicking in the streets, law and order breaking down, the playing of loud and licentious music, egg yolks and meat pies consumed in public places…

But you know, it is not only in the elderly that a low-cholesterol diet is associated with a higher mortality rate. The Austrians carried out a study of 149,650 men and women, looking at cholesterol levels and cardiovascular and all-cause mortality. It was entitled: 'Why Eve is not Adam: prospective follow-up in 149,650 women and men of cholesterol and other risk factors related to cardiovascular and all-cause mortality'. This study lasted 15 years and looked at nearly 70,000 men, and more than 80,000 women ranging from 20 to 95 years of age who underwent, between them, more than 450,000 examinations. This was a huge study. One of the biggest and longest ever. And I am willing to bet a large sum of money that you have never heard of it.

One of the reasons for this is that it ended up being published in the *Journal of Women's Health*. Not that I have anything against this journal – how could I? I had never heard of it before tracking down this study. But why was this not published in the *BMJ*, or *The Lancet* or the *New England Journal of Medicine?* It was of huge public-health significance, yet it ended up in a journal with a relatively low 'impact' factor and was thus, effectively, buried.

However, what this study confirmed is that a low cholesterol level after the age of 50 (and under 50, if you are a man) is significantly associated with all-cause mortality:

> *In men, across the entire age range… and in women from the age of 50 onward only, low cholesterol was significantly associated with all-cause mortality, showing significant associations with death through cancer, liver diseases, and mental diseases.*

You can't get clearer than that. If you have a low cholesterol level, you are at a much greater risk of death.

Perhaps you would prefer a British study? This from the *BMJ* in 1995:

> *Low serum cholesterol concentrations (<4.8mmol/l), present in 5% of the men, were associated with the highest mortality from all causes, largely due to a significant increased in cancer deaths.*

Or perhaps you would like a Finnish study? This was a report produced 25 years into the Seven Countries Study, published in the *American Journal of Epidemiology* in 1992:

> *During the first ten years of follow-up… men with high cholesterol levels had lower all-cause mortality… because of their low cancer mortality and residual mortality.*

What about a study in the very old? The oldest old – those over 85. The following was published in *The Lancet* in 1998:

> *Each 1mmol/l increase in total cholesterol corresponded to a 15% decrease in mortality.*

Or how about this one from France, published in *The Lancet* in 1989? A small study, admittedly, but quite amazing nonetheless. Ninety-two women living in a nursing home, most of whom died over the next five years. The lowest mortality rate was at an average cholesterol level of 7.0mmol/l, and the highest mortality rate was at an average cholesterol level of 4.0mmol/l. At this level, the mortality rate was 5.2 times higher than at 7.0mmol/l. You probably thought that anyone with a cholesterol level of seven had died fifty years earlier of a heart attack. Not so.

Enough already, I hear you cry. OK, enough already. I shall merely summarise the data on overall mortality:

- Under the age of 50, your cholesterol level doesn't really make much difference to your risk of dying. However, if your cholesterol level starts falling, watch out. You are at a terrible risk – a 429 per cent increased risk of death per 1mmol/l cholesterol drop, according to the Framingham Study.

- After the age of 50, a low cholesterol level is associated with a significantly greater overall mortality. The older you get, the more dangerous it is to have a low cholesterol level.

Does this mean that a low cholesterol level is, itself, deadly? No, I don't think so. I do not believe that a low or a high cholesterol/LDL level actually causes anything except, perhaps, haemorrhagic stroke – if the level is very low. I think it is mainly a disease 'marker' of a kind. Although, in general, it seems much more dangerous to have a low level than a high level.

Of course, I am not the only person in the world to have noticed that low cholesterol levels are associated with increased mortality. The mainstream research community also picked up on this one. Perhaps, to be more accurate, I should say the mainstream research community has failed to sweep this fact under the carpet. (Or maybe they have, since no one I speak to is ever aware of this fact.) What is their explanation? It is as follows. A falling, or low cholesterol level, is a sign of an underlying disease. Thus it is not the low cholesterol level that kills you, it is the underlying disease.

It is true that certain diseases – e.g. advanced cancer – can create a low cholesterol level, as can liver diseases such as chronic Hepatitis B. This makes it likely that some people with low cholesterol levels are suffering from a serious underlying disease. Therefore, this is one ad-hoc hypothesis with which I am in a certain amount of agreement.

The leading proponent of this hypothesis is a researcher called Carlos Iribarren. I think he was the first to propose the idea that a low cholesterol level indicates underlying disease, and he bangs on about it regularly. Whether it was his original idea or not, the rest of the scientific community fell upon this concept gratefully, and now repeat it as their new mantra. Thus, everyone can reassure themselves with the knowledge that a raised cholesterol really, truly, is deadly. Even when it's low – perhaps especially when it's low.

Time to quote from one of Iribarren's studies, published in the *Journal of the American Medical Association* (JAMA). This study was designed to prove that a low cholesterol level was not an independent risk factor for death. The conclusion of the study:

> *We conclude that the excess mortality at low TC [total cholesterol] levels can be partially explained by confounding with other determinants of death and by pre-existing disease at baseline… In our study TC level was not associated with increased cancer or all-cause mortality in the absence of smoking, high alcohol consumption, and hypertension.*

So there you go. Once you add in smoking, high alcohol consumption and high blood pressure, you find that low cholesterol levels disappear as a risk factor.

Now, I was explaining that, according to mainstream researchers, a low cholesterol level is not a risk factor for dying, because it is, in turn, caused by an underlying disease, and it's the underlying disease that kills you – not the low cholesterol level. Maybe in some cases this is true. However, I find the idea that cancer can cause a low cholesterol level – before the cancer can even be detected – somewhat bizarre.

An early stage cancer is smaller than a grain of rice – far smaller. The possibility that 0.1g, or thereabouts, of tumour mass can have a discernible effect on cholesterol levels seems utterly bizarre. How could it? Of course, when you have advanced cancer, this knackers the entire metabolic system. But can cancer do this five or ten years before diagnosis? I think I will go as far as to say that this is impossible.

In fact, I don't need to rely on such theoretical arguments, because this ad-hoc hypothesis has actually been disproved. The Framingham research team had also noted a high mortality rate in over-50s who had low cholesterol levels. They too wondered if the low cholesterol levels were caused by an underlying illness:

> *Similar results from several modified analyses make low cholesterol levels due to a severe illness an unlikely explanation for our results.*

Sorry about that tortured passage, but I do try to use the exact words of the researchers, rather than put my words in their mouths. (For some reason, people seem to find this more believable.) However, I shall translate. Those with low cholesterol levels did not have a severe underlying illness. They just had long-term low cholesterol levels followed by a much higher mortality rate. And however many 'modified analyses' were used, they just couldn't sweep this association under the carpet without leaving a big bump sticking up in the middle.

The Honolulu researchers also looked carefully at their findings in the light of the Iribarren ad-hoc hypothesis:

> *Iribarren and colleagues suggested that a decline in serum cholesterol might occur over a decade before diagnosis of a disease [yeah, right – my words], and such long-term morbidity could be attributable to chronic subclinical infections with Hepatitis B, or to chronic respiratory diseases.*
>
> *... our data suggest that those individuals with a low serum cholesterol maintained over a twenty-year period will have the worst outlook for all cause mortality.*
>
> *Our present analysis suggest that this [Iribarren's] hypothesis is implausible and is unlikely to account for the adverse effects of low cholesterol levels over twenty years.*

This is as close as one set of researchers will ever come to telling another set of researchers that they are talking complete bollocks. At least in public, anyway.

Just to ram home the point, the Austrian researchers also analysed their data to see if underlying diseases caused the low cholesterol levels:

> *For the first time, we demonstrate that the low cholesterol effect occurs even among younger respondents, contradicting the previous assessments among cohorts of older people that this is a proxy or marker for frailty occurring with age.*

In a way, it's a shame. I rather like Iribarren's hypothesis in a kind of last-desperate-throw-of-the-dice kind of a way. Low cholesterol levels are caused by early stage diseases, so early that you can't actually detect them. So how do we know they are there? Well we can't, obviously… duh! They're undetectable, stupid. But we know they must be there, otherwise these people wouldn't have low cholesterol levels. Yes, it's the good old circular argument again.

Q: 'Why have these people got low cholesterol levels?'
A: 'Because of an underlying disease.'
Q: 'How do you know they have an underlying disease?'
A: 'Well, just look at the low cholesterol levels. They couldn't have such a low level if they did not have an underlying disease.'

What I find perhaps most amusing about this area is the 'clash of the mighty ad-hoc hypotheses'. On one hand we have Iribarren explaining that a low cholesterol level is caused by underlying diseases. So a low cholesterol level is a sign of being completely knackered. On the other hand, we have another group of researchers – led by the mighty Law and Wald, quelle surprise – explaining that 'primitive' peoples have very, very low levels of blood cholesterol, and this is exceedingly healthy. 'You cannot have a cholesterol level that is too low. Statinate, statinate!'

So a low cholesterol level in the West is a sign of desperate illness, but a low cholesterol level among primitive peoples is a sign of glowing health – something we should all aspire to achieve. Go figure, as they say. I say, go look at the life expectancy of primitive peoples and then tell me how healthy a low cholesterol level might be. 'Oh, but they have such a high mortality rate because they die of things other than heart disease.' (Well they would, wouldn't they – see everything written above.)

Maybe all groups of researchers should get together and try to put together a story that doesn't keep contradicting itself all the time. Fat chance. To be honest, I don't think that they are even aware that they are arguing directly against each other in their attempts to defend the cholesterol hypothesis. One lot are digging a hole, and the others are frantically filling it in again. Still, it's probably good for the GDP.

Moving on from Iribarren, and all the other desperate ad-hoc hypotheses that I really don't have time to mention, the simple fact is this: a low cholesterol level increases the risk of death in men and women. This is one fact that has never been contradicted by any study. It is also a fact that is so well hidden that no one I have ever spoken to is aware of it. Indeed, when I mention it, no one actually believes me.

It is also rather important. The fact that a low cholesterol level is unhealthy may even make you think about your cholesterol level in a whole new way. Is it around 5.5mmol/l and above? Good. Below 4.0mmol/l? Watch out.

WOMEN AND HEART DISEASE

Now it is time to look directly at cholesterol levels and heart disease. I will start by looking at women and heart disease, an area of research that may otherwise be referred to as 'The case of the mysterious disappearing fact' starring female sex hormones, the ever-popular menopause, evil LDL and our plucky hero HDL. Along with a full supporting cast of ad-hoc hypotheses – as always.

It has been recognised for many years that women, generally, suffer much less heart disease than men – especially younger women. The difference is normally about 300 per cent. This is despite the fact that women have higher average cholesterol levels. The widest gap I found was in New Zealand in the 1970s. Here, women aged 45–55 had one-tenth the mortality rate of men. Now that's what I call a gap.

Women, therefore, present a problem for the cholesterol hypothesis. Higher cholesterol levels than men, but much lower rates of heart disease. This must mean that…

Eager schoolboy: 'Sir, sir… it must mean that raised cholesterol levels don't cause heart disease.'
Teacher: 'You stupid boy. We know that raised cholesterol levels cause heart disease. Anybody else?'
Teacher's pet: 'It means that women must be protected against a high cholesterol level, sir.' (Smug grin.)
Teacher: 'Well done, Snodgrass, that is the correct answer.'

At this point it is worth presenting some data. These data come, once again, from 1992 and the 'Report of the Conference on Low Blood Cholesterol: Mortality Associations', published in *Circulation*. The researchers looked at all available data on women from 11 major studies or trials, representing 124,818 women. Their conclusions:

> *Many findings for women were discrepant from those for men. Of particular importance in women was considered to be the essentially flat relation of total cholesterol to total mortality, total cardiovascular, and total cancer mortality.*

See graph oveleaf (Fig. 25).

Yes, it's the *female* paradox.

Don't worry, you see this is not actually a paradox. ('Phew, for a minute there you had me worried.') Women, you see, are protected against a raised cholesterol level by their sex hormones. Ad-hoc hypothesis no. 8,396,249.

For many years, I too, believed that women were protected by their sex hormones. Everyone said it, everyone believed it. After all,

Fig. 25 Risk of cardiovascular death at different cholesterol levels – women

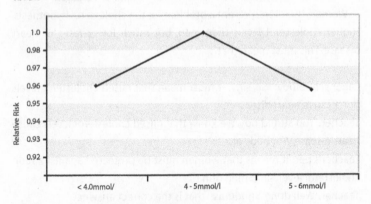

protection disappeared after the menopause, doesn't it? I'm sure I've read that many times.

Well, in 1963, a study was carried out on women who had had hysterectomies. Half of the women had their ovaries removed at the same time – thus they had no sex hormones – and half retained their ovaries. (I think I should make it clear that the removal, or retention, of the ovaries was done purely on medical need; if not, this would have been one of the world's least ethical studies…)

The results:

> We found no difference in the prevalence of coronary heart disease in the oopherectomised [both ovaries removed] and hysterectomised [no ovaries removed] women.
>
> The finding of no difference in the arteriosclerotic heart disease rates in the two groups suggests that some factor, or factors, apart from ovarian function are responsible for the relative freedom from coronary heart disease in women as compared to men.

I think that this was the first time anyone actually put the sex hormone ad-hoc hypothesis to the test, and it failed utterly and completely. Of course, the results had no discernible effect on anyone, or anything.

Eyes tightly closed to the available evidence, researchers continued to study female sex hormones and the menopause – in relation to heart disease – and they continued to find the same thing:

> *The normal menopause, which causes a gradual decrease in oestrogen production, was not associated with any increase in the risk of coronary heart disease.*

That quote from the *New England Journal of Medicine* in 1987. Ten years before, a study had appeared in the *BMJ* that looked at heart disease in relation to age, sex and the menopause:

> *… nevertheless, the idea of male sex hormones putting men at extra risk is more plausible than that of female sex hormones being protective, since large doses of oestrogen given to men for prostatic cancer, and the use of oral contraceptives containing oestrogen and progesterone have been shown to increase the risk of dying from coronary heart disease… Furthermore, the idea that female sex hormones protect against coronary heart disease should probably be abandoned.*

In fact, there has never been a study – ever – showing that female sex hormones protect against heart disease in humans. Depressingly, however, without the slightest scrap of data to feed on, this hypothesis managed to gain power and credence. It's the 'Blob' analogy again: 'Mere facts have no effect on the sex-hormone hypothesis! Run for the hills before we are all engulfed!' – or should that be 'enblobbed'?

Indeed, so powerful did the sex-hormone ad-hoc hypothesis become that, by the 1990s, millions of women were actively being prescribed hormone replacement therapy (HRT) to reduce the risk of heart disease. Several GP colleagues mutter and go red when I mention this to them. Others have wiped their memory banks of ever having done such a thing. 'Does not compute, does not compute. I was merely trying to prevent osteoporosis.'

So what changed? What changed was that someone finally decided to put the sex-hormone hypothesis to the test in a proper, grown-up, clinical trial: the heart and estrogen/progestin study – or HERS. This was randomised, placebo-controlled, and all those other things that can actually prove, or disprove, a causal relationship rather than relying solely on teleoanalysis.

I think you can guess the results by now – if you didn't know them already. Basically, HRT increases the rate of heart disease. As of today, the American Heart Association, a bastion of conventional thinking, recommends strongly against using HRT to protect against heart disease.

How many women died from heart disease having been prescribed HRT? I only ask in the spirit of disinterested scientific discovery. I would never dream of suggesting that any advice given by the 'establishment' could possibly ever have been harmful. Opinion leaders are infallible, don'tcha know.

In fact, I think the idea that female sex hormones protect against heart disease represents, possibly, the most perfect example of the pure ad-hoc hypothesis in the history of medicine. It came into existence for one reason, and one reason only. To provide an explanation for the alleged female 'protection' against raised cholesterol levels. It was based on no evidence whatsoever. In fact, every time it was studied it was disproved, yet it still failed to die. It was only a very large, controlled clinical study that finally killed it.

Now that it is dead, what is left to account for female protection? My explanation is as follows:

A high cholesterol level does not cause heart disease. It is caused by other things. Which means that there is no need to ask why women are protected against high cholesterol levels, because, you see, there is nothing from which to be protected.

And wouldn't accepting this possibility make life easier?

If there is no connection between cholesterol levels and heart disease, then there is no need to try and explain why, as cholesterol levels rose in Japan, the rate of heart disease fell. There is no need to explain why women have a lower rate of heart disease than men, despite having higher cholesterol levels. Because there is nothing to explain.

But if you accept this interpretation of the facts, you have just destroyed the cholesterol hypothesis. And that would never do. 'Off with his head,' bellowed the Queen of Hearts. And so another ad-hoc hypothesis was rapidly wheeled into place – one that had been prepared earlier. 'You see, my dear boy, it never was female sex hormones that protected women as I, ahem, said all along. Instead, it is the fact that women, generally, have higher HDL levels, and this protects against heart disease.' (Ad-hoc hypothesis no. 3 billion, and counting.) To quote a study in *Geriatrics*:

> *High-density lipoproteins and triglyceride levels are independent predictors of CVD in women. Cholesterol screening guidelines should be re-evaluated to reflect the importance of HDL and triglycerides in determining CVD risk in women.*

To quote Dr Malcolm Kendrick, your author:

> *Oh for God's sake, can you not just give up and admit that you are wrong?*

Actually, the above quote from *Geriatrics* came before the HERS finally impaled the sex-hormone conjecture. Indeed, I believe the only reason why the HERS was widely accepted, rather than subjected to the usual rubbishing, is that mainstream researchers in heart disease were already jumping ship from sex hormones to HDL. Spurred on, no doubt, by the imminent arrival of HDL-raising agents – with all the lucrative 'swimming-pool-enhancing' clinical trials that would ensue.

A large part of me would rather not face the effort of chasing down this hypothesis and stomping it to death. But another part of me knows that the entire HDL 'good' cholesterol idea is in need of a serious kicking – as we used to say in Bonnie Scotland. After all, it has started to become the dominant hypothesis. 'Look deeply into my eyes... forget total cholesterol, forget LDL... think only of HDL.' Four legs good, two legs better.

What is a high density lipoprotein? It is a lipoprotein that is smaller, and denser, and contains more cholesterol, pound for pound, than any other type of lipoprotein. No one is certain where they come from, but the liver seems the most likely place.

What do they do? What are they for? They seem to be cholesterol 'scavengers'. When a cell dies, cholesterol is released and floats about in the spaces between the cells. A passing HDL molecule can 'incorporate' this floating cholesterol, then transfer it to a VLDL or LDL, from whence it can be reabsorbed back into the liver and reprocessed. This is the so-called 'reverse cholesterol transport system'.

It also seems that HDL can, through some system or other, remove excess cholesterol from within cells themselves. I'm not sure if I quite believe it, but incomprehensible tomes have been written on the subject. However, any argument in this area would require discussion of things like microtubular transcytosis – so I am not going there, however fascinating microtubular transcytosis may be.

Moving on – once HDL has hoovered up excess cholesterol, it is stimulated to transfer this cholesterol to an LDL or a VLDL by an enzyme known as lecithin cholesterol acyltransferase (LCAT). I only mention this rather arcane fact because several trials are underway on drugs designed to block LCAT, so that the HDL level will be increased. Although if you think this one through it makes absolutely no sense whatsoever. 'Let's block one of the central actions of the "reverse cholesterol transport" system, thought to protect against heart disease. That way we will have more HDL molecules in the bloodstream, but they won't be able to do anything, such as transferring cholesterol back to the liver.'

Still, with the lucrative 22-year patents starting to run out on all statins, the pharmaceutical companies desperately need another angle beyond mere LDL lowering, and raising HDL levels looks like it might hit the jackpot.

To my mind, this is all a case of history repeating itself, only this time as farce. Today, everyone firmly believes HDL to be protective, just like they believed in sex hormones yesterday. And yes, there were complex theories in place to explain all the mechanisms by which sex hormones achieved their protective effect, just as there are with HDL. Yet, as with sex hormones, how many randomised, controlled, clinical trials on raising or lowering HDL have there been? Have a wild guess. You're right. The answer is none. To put it another way – NONE! Or, to quote the *Journal of the American College of Cardiology*, January 2005:

> Epidemiologic evidence has shown that HDL-C is inversely related to coronary heart disease (CHD) risk. However, the evidence for reducing CHD risk by raising HDL-C is thin, predominantly due to the paucity of effective and safe HDL-increasing drugs.

'Thin'… that's a good scientific word. How about 'nonexistent'? That's a better one.

In this particular area, though, it is interesting to look again at the HERS. Why? Because one of the central reasons why sex hormones were thought to be protective is because they raised the HDL level. And, as expected, the HDL levels did rise in the HERS trial. One slight problem, though: as HDL levels rose, so did the risk of heart disease.

Or, to put this another way, when 'good' cholesterol levels went up, so did the risk of heart disease. Perhaps we need to redefine 'good' as 'bad'. George Orwell to the rescue again, I think. 'Freedom is slavery, war is peace, I'm a little teapot…'

What the HERS researchers found was a relatively small 3 per cent increase in heart disease risk for every 5.4mg/dl rise in HDL. Converting this to UK units, a 0.14mmol/l rise in HDL increased CHD risk by 3 per cent. On that basis, a 1mmol/l rise in HDL would increase the risk of heart disease by 21 per cent.

This, I admit, is not a very scientific calculation, and you're never really going to see a 1mmol/l rise in HDL anyway. But what the heck, mainstream researchers are allowed to use teleoanalysis, so I think I can get to use a little multiplication.

Despite these results, and however tempting it may be, I am not going to claim that HDL is damaging. Again, I think HDL is a marker of some kind. Almost certainly a marker of deranged carbohydrate metabolism, diabetes, insulin resistance and suchlike. Which means that a low HDL is, potentially, a worrying sign that something is going wrong with your metabolism. But it is only a sign, nothing else.

Of course, it is true that one key function of HDL is to transport cholesterol out of tissues and back to the liver via VLDL and LDL. But there is a huge difference between absorbing cholesterol that is floating about inside cells, or in the spaces between cells, and sucking cholesterol out of an atherosclerotic plaque.

Firstly, atherosclerotic plaques are almost universally covered over by a lining, or cap separating the plaque from the bloodstream, and this cap is impermeable to HDL. Secondly, a great deal of the cholesterol in plaque is in clefts, even crystals (how do you think Virchow recognised it 150 years ago?). It is not free and floating about inside a plaque, you would need a pneumatic drill to extract it, and I can't see HDL wielding a pickaxe to a cholesterol cleft.

Thirdly, no one has explained, or identified, any sort of mechanism by which HDL gets cholesterol out of a plaque. It just sort of… does it. Speaking personally, I always like to see some sort of plausible biological mechanism to explain why something works. But on this one we have an almost total silence. Actually, the silence is not almost total, it is total.

Yes, I know that HDL is part of the reverse cholesterol transport system. Big deal. You can babble about this process all you like, and it does not explain how an inanimate molecule penetrates a fibrous cap then sucks cholesterol from a plaque before returning, back through the fibrous cap, 'unharmed' to the bloodstream. 'The name is HDL… James HDL. Licensed to cure.'

To my mind, a good hypothesis should start with a theory as to how a thing may happen, based on a sound knowledge of physiology and biochemistry and the underlying science. But the HDL hypothesis only exists to plaster over yet another contradiction to the central cholesterol/LDL hypothesis. It's not really a hypothesis, it's really just an excuse, disguised as science.

However, my objections to the HDL hypothesis are not just theoretical. Now I shall introduce you to another black swan. 'A black swan,' did I hear you say? Oh yes indeedy. You see, there are two basic schools of thought in scientific research. There are the 'weight of evidence' scientists who seem to believe that if, for example, you find a high HDL level and a low rate of heart disease in ten studies, and a high HDL level yet a high rate of heart disease in two studies, you should place your faith in the ten studies. Such people are what I would call scientific 'democrats': whichever finding is supported by the greatest number of studies is the winner.

My view, and in this I am a follower of Karl Popper, is that such people are not truly scientists. The true scientific method is to propose a hypothesis in such a way that it can be refuted. You then set up experiments designed to refute the hypothesis. If you can't, the hypothesis is likely to be correct. But if you can find a refutation, the hypothesis is wrong. And it doesn't matter how many positive studies you have, they are all trumped by one contradictory study.

To use an example from Popper. A biologist offers the conjecture that all swans are white. If a black swan is discovered, his conjecture is wrong, and it doesn't matter how many white swans there are relative to black swans. Ten to one, fifty to one, a million to one. Find one black swan and you have to accept that swans come in colours other than white. There are, of course, ways round this. To quote Popper again:

> ... *when black swans are discovered in Australia he [the biologist]*
> *says that his conjecture is not refuted. He insists that black swans*

are a new kind of bird since it is part of the defining property of a
swan that it is white.

Popper, K. Popper Selections

Anyone recognise this technique?

Anyway, black swan number one was the HERS. This showed that as HDL went up, so did the risk of heart disease. Now it is time to introduce a second and third black swan.

The second black swan was a study done in Poland and the USA ten years ago. At that time, the rate of heart disease was going up very rapidly in Poland and down in the USA. Researchers wanted to know if HDL levels might be the cause of this difference. The assumption behind the study was that the HDL levels would be high in the USA and low in Poland. Just for the record, they measured three different subtypes of HDL. (Yes, even HDL fragments into smaller and smaller fractions.) Not that it actually made any difference to the study, it just makes it considerably more difficult to understand the results.

The results:

> *In Polish subjects levels of HDL-C, HDL2, and HDL3, both*
> *unadjusted and adjusted for age and lifestyle factors, were*
> *higher than in US subjects. These differences contrast sharply*
> *with rising CHD rates in Poland and suggest either that other risk*
> *factors account for this trend or that the relationship between*
> *HDL-C and CHD risk may differ between the two countries.*

In short, Polish men have high HDL levels and a high rate of heart disease.

In Russia, we find our third black swan:

> *High density lipoprotein (HDL) cholesterol was inversely related to*
> *mortality in US women, but there was no association of HDL*
> *cholesterol with mortality in Russian women. The absence of an*

association between HDL cholesterol and mortality in the Russian
sample should be investigated further.

American Journal of Epidemiology,
15 February 1994; 139(4): 369–79

Are these studies, plus the HERS, enough to demolish the hypothesis that HDL protects against CHD? In my opinion the answer is yes. If your hypothesis is that HDL protects against CHD and you can find, without trying too hard, three pieces of directly contradictory data, then your hypothesis has just been shot dead.

Or has it? For if I have discovered one thing about this area, it is that HDL protection hypothesis truly cannot be killed. For example, a community in Italy was discovered with very low HDL levels and yet a very low of heart disease:

> *Thirty years ago, researchers showed that a family living in a*
> *northern Italian town, Limone sul Garda, lived to be very old and*
> *were extraordinarily resistant to heart attacks. Lots of people live*
> *to be one hundred years old and do not suffer heart attacks, but*
> *these people were extremely unusual because they had*
> *extremely low blood levels of the good HDL cholesterol that*
> *prevents heart attacks...*

> *http://www.drmirkin.com/heart/3044.html*

So, here we have a group with low HDL levels and low rates of heart disease, yet this fact had no impact on the 'protective HDL' hypothesis. In fact, it has actually managed to strengthen it. That noise you can hear is me beating my head against a wall.

HDL protects against heart disease – check. We find a population with a very low HDL level – check. They don't die of heart disease – check. This is the strongest proof ever that HDL protects against heart disease – check.

I'm a little teapot – check...

Short and stout – check...

But hey! How silly of me to question this. You see, it has now been established that these people have a super-special form of HDL known as ApoA-1 Milano, no less. A stylish, two-door coupé form of HDL with that indefinable Italian flair and high performance. And it's protective, even at low levels – in fact, especially at low levels. Once again, low has become today's new high.

Researchers have now taken ApoA-1 Milano, cloned it in a laboratory, and started infusing it into people with heart disease, claiming results of such magnificent wonderfulness that the Emperor himself is going to clothe himself in them.

You know what? I really wouldn't hold my breath waiting for this wonder cure. Remember that ApoA-1 Milano represents an ad-hoc hypothesis that only exists because of a previous ad-hoc hypothesis, which only exists because of an ad-hoc hypothesis prior to that. I am referring to the following:

- Raised LDL is supposed to cause CHD – but not in women.
- Women have higher HDL levels – so HDL is hypothesised to be protective against raised LDL.
- A population was found with low HDL levels and low rates of heart disease – so their HDL is hypothesised to be super-protective – even at low concentrations

Thus, a whole new branch of medicine opens up. And do you know how many people from the small Italian village of Limone sul Garda this protective HDL research is based on? Thirty-eight!

ApoA-1 Milano was patented by Esperion therapeutics, and the study on this form of HDL was done by Steven Nissen who is a research collaborator with Dr Eric Topol. Topol, in turn, runs a major cardiovascular website, called www.theheart.org entirely pharma-ceutical company sponsored.

And what did the www.theheart.org have to say about the ApoA-1 Milano study?

Who would believe that with five weeks of therapy we could actually remove significant quantities of plaque from the coronaries?

Please remember that this research was non-randomised, and conducted by professionals working closely with pharmaceutical companies.

*****

Anyhow. At this point I shall attempt to summarise the evidence on HDL. What is the evidence to support the fact that HDL is protective?

- People with high HDL levels tend to have a lower rate of heart disease. And that's it.

What is the evidence against?
- In the HERS – the only study done in which proper outcomes were measured, e.g. death from heart disease – when HDL levels went up so did the rate of heart disease.
- You can find populations with a high HDL level and a high rate of heart disease, and vice versa.
- It is clear that HDL levels reflect other things, e.g. alcohol consumption, which do have a direct effect on heart disease.

What's the most important fact?
- No controlled, randomised study has even been done in which raising HDL levels has reduced the rate of heart disease.

In short, HDL should be relegated to the same status as female sex hormones. It's an ad-hoc hypothesis, pure and simple. Which is kind of critical to the female heart-disease discussion. Because once you remove HDL from the equation, there is nothing left to explain the alleged protection that women have against heart disease.

This is just as well, really. For I am now going to present evidence that women are not actually protected against a high cholesterol level at all. Women, even young women, can suffer the same rate of heart disease as men, if not higher. Yet another little-known fact.

At this point I think it would be interesting to compare British women with French men. I know they live in different countries, but so what? Why should that matter? Unless, of course, you think that the French are 'genetically protected against heart disease'. In which case you should beat yourself with a large club and dismiss yourself from the discussion.

Or perhaps you think that risk factors cannot be compared between different countries? If not, why not? If, as we are endlessly informed, cholesterol levels, blood pressure, smoking, saturated-fat consumption, age and sex are the most important risk factors for heart disease in the UK and the US, then why not in France? He who lives by the risk factor should also be prepared to die by the risk factor.

Now, if we do compare the countries we can see that firstly, French men eat more saturated fat. They also have marginally higher cholesterol levels, a greater percentage have hypertension, and French men also smoke considerably more than British women. (See table below, featuring the most recent figures from MONItor Trends in CArdiovascular Disease – or MONICA.) These are considered the critical risk factors by the major medical organisations, and they are used to calculate your risk of heart disease (along with age and sex, which are cancelled out in this comparison).

RISK FACTOR	BRITISH WOMEN	FRENCH MEN
Saturated fat % total calories	13.6%	15.5%
% with systolic BP >160mmHg	7%	11%
Total cholesterol level	5.6mmol/l	5.7mmol/l
Percentage who smoke	25	31

Yet, if we look at heart-disease rates (ages 35–74 per 100,000/year), every ten years since 1968, when statistics first started, they are as follows:

Year	CHD rate British Women	CHD rate French Men
1968	175	152
1978	180	154
1988	156	118
1998	97	85

Quelle horreur! French men have a lower rate of death from heart disease than British women, and always have done, despite having higher cholesterol levels and a greater burden of other 'risk factors'. What does this mean? What indeed.

If you want a more spectacular example of the lack of female protection, we can look at Russian women and British men:

	Russian women	**British men**
Rate of smoking	10%	27%
Average cholesterol levels	5.4mmol/l	6.0mmol/l
Average systolic BP	132	134
Saturated-fat consumption	8.2% of calories	13.6% of calories
Death rate from heart disease (200)	267/100,000/year	229/100,00/year

As you can see, British men smoke almost three times as much as Russian women, they have 10 per cent higher cholesterol levels, slightly higher blood pressure and eat 40 per cent more saturated fat. And yet their heart disease rate is 14 per cent lower.

At this point I think I should highlight the fact that French men have far more risk factors than Russian women, and 300 per cent less heart disease. What the HDL is going on?

You may feel that it is unscientific for me to make comparisons between different countries (although I would be interested to hear your reasoning). If so, I shall look within the same countries.

In Brazil, in 1989, women suffered a higher rate of heart disease than men. Admittedly, this was the only year when women had a higher rate. However, in general, the difference between men and women in Brazil is, and remains, tiny. Below are their respective risk factors:

Risk Factor	Brazilian Men	Brazilian women
% with hypertension	19	27
Average cholesterol level	4.92 mmol/l	5.10 mmol/l
% who smoke	24	18
% who are obese	48	39

OK, so their risk factors are pretty similar. But then again, risk factors for men and women are pretty similar in most countries. Yet, on average, women have one-third the rate of heart disease. In fact in the UK it is one-third, in France it is one-quarter. In New Zealand, at one point, it was one-tenth. In Brazil there is no difference.

But I am not going to stop here, because there are countries where women suffer more heart disease than men. For example, an Indian study in Delhi in 1993 showed that:

- The overall incidence of CHD was 19.7 per 1,000
- Men: 17.3 per 1,000
- Women: 21.0 per 1,000

In New Zealand in the 1970s, it was found that Maori women had more than twice the rate of heart disease of men, as revealed in a study in the *New Zealand Medical Journal*:

> *This paper reports the prevalence of coronary heart disease (CHD) and its relationship with several standard risk factors in samples of New Zealand Maoris… The prevalence rates of CHD are: 16.1 percent, and 7.3 percent in Maori females and males respectively.*

Confused yet? If so, I would like to state that this is really not my fault.

I think everything is quite simple, it's the endless ad-hoc hypotheses developed to protect the cholesterol hypothesis that have created this current unholy mess of sex hormones, HDL, ApoA-1 Milano and their like.

In the end, to cut through the confusion, you have to take this argument down to basics. Women are either protected against a high cholesterol level or they are not. If women are protected against a high cholesterol level, how can you explain the fact that there are populations where women have lower cholesterol levels than men, yet suffer more heart disease? Where is the protection here? Where's it gone?

On the other hand, if women are not protected against a high cholesterol level, why do they have much less heart disease than men – in most countries – when they have higher cholesterol levels? Run these arguments any way you like, and they keep breaking down as logic snaps under the strain.

In fact, there is only one conclusion that can be drawn from this unholy mess: cholesterol levels have no effect on heart disease rates in women. No other explanation fits the facts, but this explanation fits perfectly without the need for any ad-hoc hypothesis. Or, indeed, any other explanation at all. Remove cholesterol from the equation and all confusion disappears. Simple, isn't it?

You might then ask, well, why do women generally get much less heart disease than men? That, of course, is the $64,000 question, and one that I shall answer in due course.

RAISED CHOLESTEROL LEVELS AND HEART DISEASE IN MEN

At this point, things are beginning to thin out somewhat. A raised cholesterol level doesn't cause strokes, but a low cholesterol level may well do. A raised cholesterol level doesn't increase overall mortality, but a low cholesterol level does. A raised cholesterol level does not cause heart disease in women.

What's left? Does a raised cholesterol level cause heart disease in men?

Here are two facts with which I fully agree.

1: In men under the age of 50, a raised cholesterol level is associated with an increased risk of heart disease. (Note that I didn't say 'caused', I said 'associated'.)

2: Within countries/populations, a higher cholesterol level in men is associated with a higher rate of heart disease.

Does this mean that a high blood-cholesterol level causes heart disease in men? I dinnae think so, laddie. You see, there is far, far too much directly contradictory evidence out there.

Time, I think, to introduce you to Australian Aboriginal men for the first time. This group has one of the highest – possibly *the* highest – rates of heart disease in the world. They have a rate that currently stands at 1,100 per 100,000/year. This is about four times the rate in the UK, and more than ten times the rate in France. (It is a stunning 50 times the rate in French women.)

The average blood-cholesterol level in Aboriginal men is 4.9mmol/l, contrasting with 6.1mmol/l in the UK. Their average blood pressure is 125/77 – considerably lower than men in the UK. Their average HDL level is 1.1mmol/l, which is 0.2mmol/l lower than the UK. Their average body mass index (BMI) is 23.2, which makes them considerably less obese than British men.

The only conventional risk factor where they truly lead the way is smoking, which stands at just over 80 per cent. (Slightly higher than the rate in Japan where, incidentally, the rate of heart disease is 20 times lower. That's right, 20 times.)

The main reason for bringing up the Australian Aboriginals is to compare and contrast their rate of heart disease, and average cholesterol levels, with countries from the MONICA study discussed previously. This study has been going on for ages now. It was set up by the WHO to look at heart disease rates and risk factors around the world.

I am a big fan of the MONICA study, by the way. It generates huge volumes of data that can be relied upon to be accurate and objective. So three cheers to the WHO. The interpretation of their data may often be exceedingly dodgy, but the data themselves are trustworthy. MONICA is where I found the data on saturated fat consumption across Europe.

For years, MONICA can remain silent then, every so often, it bestirs itself and out plops a golden egg. One of the latest golden eggs came from its review of cholesterol levels across Europe. I related these data to its published death rates from heart disease. And to this list I have added in the Australian Aboriginals and drawn a graph (Fig.26):

Fig. 26 Comparison between heart-disease rates in men aged 35–74 and average cholesterol levels in 15 populations

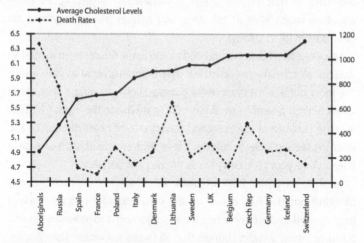

As you can see, ahem, a very clear pattern emerges. As average cholesterol levels rise heart disease rates fall, then go up, then fall, then go up, then fall, then fall a bit more, then go up, then fall. I suppose the general trend is that as cholesterol levels rise, heart-disease rates fall. But I would not even attempt to make such a claim from that graph.

The point I want to make is that there is a complete and utter dissociation between cholesterol levels and heart disease. And no, I didn't choose these countries to make my point. I just took all the countries that appeared on page 77 of the European cardiovascular disease statistics from the WHO MONICA Project:

Mean total blood cholesterol and percentage with levels of 6.5mmol/l and above, adults aged 35–64, by sex, latest available data, MONICA Project populations. [NB: I only used data on men in this graph.]

This was published in the *International Journal of Epidemiology*. Go look it up if you don't believe me. The only countries I left out are Yugoslavia and East Germany, which <u>were</u> in the most recent MONICA statistics available on cholesterol levels – somewhat surprising, as these countries didn't exist at the time, and neither did any statistics on deaths from heart disease.

I suppose that I didn't really need to add in the figures from Australian Aboriginals to make my point. But they represent, as far as I am aware, the most outrageous cholesterol 'paradox'. Lowest average cholesterol levels, highest rate of heart disease. Compare this to the Swiss – highest average cholesterol levels, second lowest rate of heart disease. Or the Russians, second lowest cholesterol level, highest rate of heart disease in Europe. Take your pick. Every single country is a 'paradox'.

And so, an entire flock of black swans wheels overhead, nearly blocking out the sun. Below us, the cardiovascular opinion leaders eagerly tend to their one white swan, subjecting it to intense scientific scrutiny. 'I think we can confirm that all swans are white.' They intone. 'Could someone please shoot those strange black birds above us; they are distracting us from our work.'

Somewhat closer to home are 'Emigrant Asian Indians'. The term is not mine, and it is rather confusing. Emigrant Asian Indians, in the context of heart-disease research, means anyone who emigrates from Pakistan, India, Sri Lanka and/or Bangladesh. It has been known for years that Emigrant Asians, as I shall call them, suffer catastrophically high rates of heart disease. This is true wherever they emigrate to.

And what of their risk factors for heart disease? A study in Bradford, looking at 'Ethnic differences in risk markers for heart disease in Asian immigrants', found that, in comparison to the surrounding non-Asian population:

- They had lower total cholesterol levels
- They had lower LDL levels
- They had lower blood pressure
- They smoked less
- They were slightly less obese

So there you have it. The reason why Asian Indians in the UK have higher rates of heart disease is because they have lower LDL and total cholesterol levels, smoke less and have lower blood pressure. A study of Emigrant Asian Indians in the USA came to the following conclusions:

> *Asian Indians have the highest rates of coronary artery disease (CAD) of any ethnic group studied, despite the fact that nearly half of this group are life-long vegetarians [my emphasis]. CAD occurs early in age and generally follows a malignant course, although the incidence of classic risk factors is low.*
>
> *Enas A Clin Cardiol, March 1995*

In more detail, the figures from Asian Indians in the USA were as follows:

Risk Factor	Asian Indians	Caucasians
Rate of obesity	4.2%	22.6%
Rate of Hypertension	14.2%	19.1%
Percentage with high LDL	13.7%	22.3%
Smoking rate	1.3%	27.1%

Different country, same findings. But of course (sound of me slapping my forehead in the background) Asian Indians are genetically susceptible to developing diabetes, and diabetes causes a huge increase in the rate of heart disease. How silly of me to forget. So what you're saying is that Australian Aboriginals and Asian Indians must have descended from the same gene pool. That famous prehistoric group of 'diabetics who drop dead of heart disease while having low cholesterol levels'. Caused by a gene found on chromosome twelve.

The descendants of this genetic line, then, must also have fought their way across the Pacific to North America, because another major population that has low cholesterol levels and a catastrophically high rate of heart disease are Native Americans. Look up the 'Strong Heart Study' on the internet. They sure get about, these 'low-cholesterol high-heart-disease offspring', considering how young they die.

If we are tracing genetic trees, I suppose we need to include Russia, because a major study was done in Russia in response to the rapid rise of heart disease-related deaths during the latter half of the 20th century. It was called 'Increased risk of coronary heart disease death in men with low total and low density lipoprotein cholesterol in the Russian Lipid Research Clinics Prevalence Follow-up Study'. If you want to look it up, the main author of the report was Shestov, of the Institute of Experimental Medicine, Russian Academy of Medical Sciences, St Petersburg. As you can see from the title, Shestov discovered that in Russia, in a significant number of men, a low LDL level was the most important risk factor for dying of heart disease:

*The results disclose a sizeable subset of **hypo**cholesterolaemics [my emphasis] in the population at increased risk of cardiac death.*

So, Australian Aboriginals, Native Americans, Emigrant Asian Indians and a large percentage of Russian men have low cholesterol levels and high rates of heart disease. Hmmm. And the Swiss and the French have very high cholesterol levels and very low rates of heart disease. Who's next? What's next?

What's next, I think, is to make the following point. Heart disease is primarily a disease of older people. The rate of heart disease in 65-year-old men is approximately 10 times that of 45-year-old men. Yet, while a raised cholesterol level is associated with heart disease in younger men, the association disappears as men get older. Here is a summary of the findings of a study published in the *Journal of the American Medical Association* in 1995:

> *Our findings do not support the hypothesis that hyper-cholesterolemia or low HDL-C are important risk factors for all-cause mortality, coronary heart disease mortality, or hospitalization for myocardial infarction or unstable angina in this cohort of persons older than 70 years.*

This is supported by another study published in the *Journal of the American Geriatric Society* in 1991:

> *Elevated total cholesterol was **not** found to be associated with CHD mortality in older men.*

And just for luck, here's another one from the National Centre for Health Statistics:

> *Although coronary heart disease remains a leading cause of death and disability in old age, the relationship of serum cholesterol level to risk of coronary heart disease in old age is controversial. Data for 2,388 white persons aged 65–74... were examined to determine the relationship of serum cholesterol level to coronary heart disease incidence... there was no overall relationship between serum cholesterol level and coronary heart disease risk in either men or women...*

How can a risk factor for a disease stop being a risk factor at the age when the disease kills the greatest number of people? What on earth is the reasoning here? That raised cholesterol levels only do damage when people are younger? Actually, I have yet to hear an explanation for this. It's another fact that is just quietly swept under the carpet, as if it were of minimal importance.

But it is critical. This would be like finding that smokers suffer an increased risk of lung cancer at 45, but by the time they are 65, smoking ceases to be a risk factor – so you might as well keep on puffing away. How much sense would that make? That's right, it would make no sense at all...

Hold on. Unless... unless a high cholesterol level didn't actually cause heart disease, but just acted as a heart-disease 'marker' in younger men. Yes, that would make sense. Hmmm.

* * * * *

At this point I should remind you of the data from the Framingham Study demonstrating that if your cholesterol level falls, your rate of cardiovascular disease increases:

> ... there is a direct association between falling cholesterol levels over the first 14 years [of the study] and mortality over the following 18 years (11% overall and 14% CVD death rate increase per 1mg/dl per year drop in cholesterol levels).

So, a falling cholesterol level causes strokes and heart disease? How does that work, then? Maybe a falling cholesterol level drags the arteries down with it? Perhaps the discussion should just stop here as I draw together the salient facts:

- A raised cholesterol level is associated with heart disease in younger men – within a country.
- There is no association at all between average cholesterol levels and the heart disease rate between countries.
- Over the age of about 50, the association between cholesterol levels and heart disease disappears.

- A falling cholesterol level is associated with a greater risk of heart disease.

If you are not convinced by now that raised cholesterol levels do not cause heart disease, nothing could possibly convince you. But before moving on to look at familial hypercholesterolaemia and such matters, I would like to introduce you to a major study that I find unintentionally hilarious.

The European Society of Cardiology runs a very major pan-European study called EUROASPIRE, which looks at risk factors for heart disease across Europe, and also analyses the management of those risk factors. A couple of years ago they found that:

> ... *smoking, previous coronary heart disease and diabetes proved significant predictors of total, cardiovascular (CVD) and coronary heart disease (CHD) mortality. Obesity, low education, **raised blood pressure, elevated total cholesterol and low HDL cholesterol** [my emphasis], however, were not significantly associated with higher mortality rates.*

But they had an explanation for the fact that raised blood pressure, raised cholesterol and low HDL cholesterol were not associated with heart-disease mortality:

> *Failure to find statistically significant associations between other classical risk factors, such as blood pressure and plasma lipid levels, and mortality may be related to the extensive use of antihypertensive and lipid-lowering drugs in this cohort.*

Perhaps they should have read the conclusion of a sister EUROASPIRE paper on the management of said risk factors:

> *This European survey of coronary patients shows a high prevalence of unhealthy lifestyles, modifiable risk factors **and***

inadequate use of drug therapies to achieve blood pressure and lipid goals [my emphasis].

The actual figures were that 58 per cent had total cholesterol concentrations over 5.5 mmol/l and more than 50 per cent had blood pressure above 150/90. In short, there was not 'extensive use of antihypertensive and lipid-lowering drugs in this cohort'. Or if there was, they weren't doing much to lower blood pressure or cholesterol levels. Another instant ad-hoc hypothesis bites the dust.

What EUROASPIRE actually proved, rather nicely, is that smoking, already having heart disease and having diabetes are true risk factors for heart disease. Whereas a high cholesterol level, and a high blood pressure, are not. Did the authors of this study consider this possibility? They did not. In this area, the ability of researchers to ignore the results of their own research is quite mind-bending.

> Men occasionally stumble over the truth, but most of them pick
> themselves up and hurry off as if nothing had happened.
>
> Winston Churchill

As a quick aside, discovering that 'already having heart disease' is a risk factor for dying of heart disease hardly ranks alongside the discovery of penicillin.

FAMILIAL HYPERCHOLESTEROLAEMIA

Enough of men and heart disease, and endless contradictions to the cholesterol hypothesis. Time now to look at a group of people who have extremely high levels of LDL in their bloodstream and who can die, aged five, of heart disease. Yes, I am talking about people with familial hypercholesterolaemia (FH).

Most doctors that I know find the evidence on FH particularly powerful and utterly convincing. It's a kind of 'A-ha!' type of fact: 'A raised cholesterol level must cause heart disease, because people with FH die very young of heart disease, and the only problem they have is a high LDL/cholesterol level. A-ha!'

And a-ha! to you too.

In fact, I sometimes think of FH as the 'Lourdes' of the cholesterol believer. 'Are you feeling dispirited? Have you too begun to feel that the cholesterol hypothesis may be falling apart? Visit Familial Hypercholesterolaemialand.

'Here you can see children with severe FH dying as young as five from heart disease. Here men and women with FH can have a 9,686 per cent increase in the risk of dying of heart disease. In Hypercholesterolaemialand, men barely make it past 40 before keeling over and dying.' Of course! How could I ever have doubted the cholesterol hypothesis? It's true, it's true!

Here, for instance, are some figures taken from the Simon Broome Register Group, set up in the UK to study and help manage people with FH:

> The cohort was followed up for 2,234 person years during 1980–9… The excess mortality from this cause (CHD) was highest at age 20–39 (standardised mortality ratio 9,686).

A 9,686 per cent increased risk of dying of heart disease! Take that! Now Dr Kendrick you must give in, abandon, buckle under, capitulate, cave in, cede, commit, concede, consign, cry uncle, deliver up, eat crow, eat dirt, entrust, fall, fold, forego, give in, go down, go under, hand over, knuckle, knuckle under, leave, let go, lump it, pack in, part with, play dead, quit, relinquish, renounce, resign, roll over, say uncle, submit, succumb, waive and yield.

I never had any intention of doing so. Because, as with everything in the strange, distorted world of the cholesterol hypothesis, facts are not exactly what they seem – even when they are true.

For instance, here is a later paper from the same Simon Broome study:

> A study showing that although mortality from heart disease is increased in FH, cancer mortality is reduced by nearly half, so that the overall mortality is no higher than in the general population of England and Wales.

So FH is a deadly killer disease, but it doesn't actually kill you. Perhaps a nigh-on 10,000 per cent increase in the risk of dying of heart disease is not exactly what you thought it was. Don't worry, it never is.

Time, I think, to reveal a little game that researchers play with statistics in the world of heart disease. It's called 'Data Inflation – the Revenge'. By the way, as you will see later, the statin researchers have taken this game to infinity – and beyond.

To give you an example of how to warp statistics into weapons of mass disinformation, I shall pose a simple question. What are the chances of winning the jackpot in the lottery? About 1 in 15 million per week. If I were able to improve your odds from 1 in 15 million to a massive 1.5 in 15 million, I could claim to have increased your chances of winning by 50 per cent. Fifty per cent, however, represents the relative increase in your chances. The absolute increase is 0.5 in 15,000,000. Or 1 in 30 million. Or, in percentage terms, 0.000003 per cent.

If I were trying to sell my lottery-enhancing service to you, which figure do you think I would use? I see an advert coming on: 'Do you want to be a MILLIONAIRE? If so, the world-renowned lottery expert and Nobel prize-winning mathematician Dr Kendrick can increase your chance of winning the lottery by 50 per cent – yes, FIFTY PER CENT! You CAN be a winner! Just send £10 in a stamped addressed envelope to the following address to receive your advice! This is NO CON TRICK, this advice is guaranteed to work.'

On the other hand, I should most likely not advertise my services thus: 'The desperate, lonely, and rather hard-up Dr Kendrick can very slightly increase your miserably small chance of winning the lottery by a meagre, and almost unnoticeable 0.000003 per cent. Yes, pitiful isn't it, you pathetic, snivelling toe-rag. But if you feel like wasting £10, send a stamped addressed envelope…'

You have to admit that 50 per cent sounds rather more impressive than 0.000003 per cent. However, both figures are true. Ah yes, the truth. A slippery little worm is it not. Oh, by the way, the best way to increase your chances of winning the lottery by 50 per cent is to buy three tickets between two people. Worth £10 of anyone's money, that advice.

To return to the Simon Broome study. In the entire population there were actually only 24 deaths, 15 of which were from heart disease. So, how many people died of heart disease in the 20–39 age group? If memory serves, it was six. From this they calculated a 9,686 per cent increase in risk. Hot dang! Aren't statistics fun? And no, I am not going to run the calculation for you. I am talking broad brush strokes here.

So while people claim massive increases in heart-disease risk with FH, the figures may not be quite what they seem – to say the least. Another reason for the overestimation of heart-disease rates in FH is that the people with FH who have been studied are the ones that already have heart disease.

> The risk of early death and premature cardiovascular disease in familial hypercholesterolaemia may have been overestimated because previous studies have looked only at patients and families who sought medical attention. Sijbrands et al traced all members of a Dutch pedigree dating from 1800 to 1989 and calculated their risk of death. They found that many untreated patients had normal life spans.
>
> http://bmj.bmjjournals.com/cgi/content/full/322/729310/b

What happened to the people with FH who did not die early of heart disease? Well, because they didn't have heart disease, no one actually knew they had FH. So the vast majority just carried on with their lives – undetected. How many such people are there? Well, difficult to tell, as they are undetected… Doh!

Luckily – for me, anyway – they are not actually always undetected. A study was done in South Africa, looking at genetic inheritance of FH. Researchers found that different members of the same family could have the gene, yet experience a very different heart-disease outcome. For example:

> One individual did not develop coronary heart disease (CHD) by age 84, despite having the FH Afrikaner-1 mutation, while his son

who inherited the same gene, developed CHD before age 50 and had to undergo bypass surgery.

So, did the FH cause premature CHD in the son? If so, why did it not cause CHD in the 84-year-old father? Same gene, same cholesterol level, completely different outcome.

At the risk of flogging a dead horse here, I would like to re-emphasise one point. If the only member of the family who had come across the medical profession had been the son, his condition would have been put down as 'yet more evidence' that FH kills people early from heart disease. The father would have slipped past unnoticed. With FH, it's a one-way evidence valve, allowing in only evidence to support your hypothesis.

Given this, do I think that FH can cause heart disease? In fact, I do. Although I believe that it is not nearly as deadly as most people believe. After all, people can live into their eighties, even nineties, and even up to 103 – in the Simon Broome study. Maybe they would have made it to 104 if they hadn't been suffering from that deadly killer FH.

However, before moving on to talk about how FH may cause heart disease, I would like to knock one thing on the head. Namely, the evidence of very early death from heart disease in homozygous FH. That is, in people who get the gene from both parents. This fact is true, but completely irrelevant to any sensible discussion.

Some years ago I was working on a medical ward when a long-term psychiatric patient was admitted. He was unconscious and very nearly died. His sodium level was 100 – which will mean nothing much to you, but we thought it was a world-record low level. Guinness World Records time indeed. Disappointingly, I then discovered lower levels. So my 15 minutes of fame have gone. What had happened to this patient? He had become very upset at the death of a friend and had started drinking water. Gallons of water. This diluted his blood to the point at which his brain nearly packed in.

I also noticed recently that drinking too much water, and then dying, is emerging as a risk factor in marathon runners who 'overhydrate', i.e. drink too much water. This from a paper in the *New England Journal of Medicine*:

> *Hyponatremia has emerged as an important cause of race-related death and life-threatening illness among marathon runners.*

Well, there you go. If you look hard enough, you can find that water is a deadly dangerous substance. And so what? Can I then argue that, because a vast excess of water is deadly, that water is deadly at any level of intake? I could try, but I don't think I would get very far.

You may remember that I mentioned Smith-Lemli-Opitz Syndrome (SLOS) earlier. This is a condition characterised by very, very low cholesterol levels, and catastrophic effects on health – stillbirth, death from multi-organ failure, visual loss, congenital heart disease and the like. This syndrome is much more deadly than FH.

Can I use the extreme example of SLOS to argue that moderately low cholesterol levels are also deadly? No, I cannot, and will not. If I did, this would be exactly the same as people claiming that premature heart disease – brought about by LDL levels in excess of 15mmol/l – somehow also provides proof that moderately raised cholesterol levels also causes heart disease.

Once you reach such extremes you are talking about a completely different pathological state. There is no substance I can think of that would not kill you if it reached five times the 'normal' level in the blood. Most things, such as sodium or potassium, will wipe you out if they vary by more than 20 per cent.

In fact, on this basis we would have to view LDL as a very benign substance indeed. You can have five times as much as normal in the bloodstream, and you can still live into your 20s, or 30s – even your 50s.

But what of more moderate FH – heterozygous FH, where LDL levels are about double normal? This still increases the rate of heart disease, although by how much I am not certain, and I don't think anyone else is either. However, even if it does, I believe that LDL may have no direct role to play.

Time now to draw the curtain aside and reveal a whole different world of research into heart disease. A world where it can be explained how FH raises the risk of dying of heart disease – but not through a raised LDL level. In another life I may have avoided talking about this world until rather later. However, I can't really say that FH raises the risk of heart disease through another mechanism, without some explanation. Otherwise, I suspect you might not believe me. Of course, you might not believe me anyway. But I rather hope that you may.

Now, let us venture into a world where researchers think that heart disease is, basically, a response to injury. The 'response to injury hypothesis' goes something like this:

- A factor (or more likely, several factors acting in unison), damages the endothelium (single-celled lining of the artery wall).
- This stimulates a small blood clot to form over the area of damage.
- Endothelium re-grows over the blood clot, 'repairing' the area of damage.
- With endothelium on top of it, the blood clot is effectively drawn into the artery wall, and is then broken down by white blood cells – thus disappearing.

That, anyway, is the healthy response to endothelial injury – if any degree of endothelial injury can actually be seen as healthy, that is. However, if the endothelium keeps getting damaged (for whatever reason), clots keep forming, and more and more blood clots keep getting drawn into the artery wall. At which point the healing responses cannot cope. The area of damage becomes permanent. A plaque forms that can grow and grow. In many cases a fibrous 'cap' forms over the plaque. This can rupture, triggering such a big blood clot that it fully blocks the artery. Heart-attack time.

That, anyway, is roughly what Austrian pathologist Carl Freiherr von Rokitansky said. And he said it more than 150 years ago. Yes, you may be surprised to learn that this is in no way a new theory. It has been around for at least as long as the cholesterol hypothesis. Perhaps even a few years longer. In fact, Rokitansky was a compatriot of Rudolf Virchow – also a man who, in my opinion, got it right. Indeed, I believe that the evidence for the 'Rokitansky' model of heart disease is overwhelming. Heart disease – or to be more accurate, 'atherosclerotic plaque formation' – is, basically, a response to injury. And it consists of two basic processes. Firstly, endothelial damage, then blood-clot formation.

As you may recall from earlier on in this book, this is exactly the research direction that Pfizer was heading off in nearly 15 years ago, before multi-billion-dollar statin profits rather distracted their attention. It is also the direction that Kilmer McCully was heading in – when he left his appointment at Harvard Medical School and Massachusetts General Hospital.

It is also the direction that Linus Pauling took for the last 20 years of his life or so. Linus Pauling is the only person, ever, to win two individual Nobel prizes. In my book, this makes him quite clever. In his later years, though, his standing within the scientific community waned as he focused increasingly on vitamin C. He claimed that it could cure just about anything, and everything. I don't believe this, but when it comes to vitamin C and heart disease he was on a very interesting track indeed. Pauling had teamed up with a certain Dr Matthias Rath on this subject. I believe Dr Rath's ideas on heart disease are brilliant. Despite a reputation for outspoken and unpopular views on anti-retroviral drugs, (which have been met with opposition from the AIDS lobby, the South African government and parts of the pharmaceutical industry), I would like to cite Dr Rath and his studies. One of Dr Rath's theories that so enamoured Linus Pauling was as follows. Humans are one of very few animal species that cannot make their own vitamin C. Included in this exclusive group are guinea pigs, fruit bats and most other large apes. Which means that the only way we humans can get sufficient vitamin C is to eat it, and we need to eat quite a lot – although perhaps not nearly as much as the two grams a day recommended by Pauling – although he did live to very nearly 100. (Maybe he had the ApoA-1 Paulingo mutation.)

If we don't eat enough vitamin C, one of the first things to happen is that our blood vessels spring leaks as the supporting collagen structure breaks down around them. Then we start to bleed, with bleeding gums being one of the early signs of scurvy. Left untreated, scurvy leads to death from internal bleeding.

It is speculated that during the ice age, our ancestors found it rather tricky to get hold of enough vitamin C, so a lot of them suffered from scurvy, and many died. However, some of them had a trick up their sleeves. This was to manufacture a lipoprotein called lipoprotein (a) – or Lp(a) – which you may remember me mentioning earlier.

Lp(a) is a form of LDL with an extra protein stuck on the side called apolipoprotein(a). This extra protein has several interesting properties. Firstly, it is attracted to areas of endothelial damage. Secondly, it sticks firmly to those areas, and helps to form a very strong and difficult-to-remove blood clot.

Thirdly, and perhaps most important of all, apolipoprotein(a) is almost identical in structure to an enzyme known as plasminogen. This enzyme is well known to the medical profession. It is incorporated into blood clots as they form. When it is activated, plasminogen turns into plasmin, and then acts like a little tiny stick of dynamite within the clot, cleaving it apart. Without plasminogen all blood clots would most likely remain in place for ever – which is not a great idea if the clot is completely blocking an artery.

Plasminogen, in turn, is activated by an enzyme known as plasminogen activator, or tissue plasminogen activator (tPA). If you are having a heart attack, you could well be given an injection of tPA to stimulate the plasminogen to blow apart the blood clot blocking your coronary arteries; tPA is thus also known as a 'clot-buster'.

Still with me? Good. Because you see, the important point here is that when Lp(a) becomes incorporated in a blood clot, it blocks the action of tPA, and makes the clot much more difficult to shift. This, of course, was probably a good thing if you were an ice-age cavemen with arteries leaking due to vitamin C deficiency. You probably needed strong 'plugs' to prevent excess blood loss, and you didn't want plasminogen blowing clots apart. But today, when no one really has vitamin C deficiency, a high level of Lp(a) may be an important factor in creating big, difficult-to-shift blood clots in your arteries. So, a high level of Lp(a) could well be a risk factor for causing the development of atherosclerotic plaques – could it not?

Of course it could. Just to give one example, a study in Spain demonstrated that people with two genes for Lp(a) expression, and high Lp(a) levels, had a 650 per cent greater risk of developing heart disease. And, increasingly Lp(a) is being isolated as an important risk factor in Emigrant Asian Indians – the ones with low LDL levels and high rates of heart disease.

I'll add one example from the Journal of Lipid Research. Rather a lengthy quote, I'm afraid, but I think it is fascinating nonetheless.

> *A high incidence of coronary heart disease (CHD) has been observed among Asian Indians immigrating to the USA and among native people remaining within the Indian subcontinent. The mortality rate for CHD in Asian Indians from Singapore is 4 times higher than in Chinese residents from Singapore, and 20 times higher than in blacks from South Africa Moreover, CHD in Asian Indians occurs prematurely and is often more severe than in Europeans…*
>
> *Traditional risk factors for CHD such as obesity, insulin-dependent diabetes mellitus, smoking, hypertension, and elevated plasma Chol or low density lipoprotein cholesterol (LDL-Chol) levels **do not** [my emphasis] explain the observed increase in CHD incidence among Asian Indians… [however, as the article goes on to say]… This study suggests that elevated plasma Lp(a) confers genetic predisposition to CHD in Asian Indians.*

By the way, forget the genetic bit, and concentrate only on the Lp(a) bit.

Finally getting back eventually to FH, is it possible that people with FH not only have high LDL levels, but that they also have high Lp(a) levels, given that they are basically the same molecule? Why, funny that you should ask. For a study was done in Austria and South Africa and the researchers found that…

This leaves little doubt that LDL-R mutations that result in FH with
elevated LDL also result in hyperlipoprotein (a).
http://atvb.ahajournals.org/cgi/content/full/20/2/522

This may all seem, I suppose, a bit theoretical. Surely people have looked at atherosclerotic plaques and found LDL within them, not Lp(a) – end of counter-hypothesis. Well, superficially at least, it seems to be true that LDL has been found in plaques, along with their key identification protein apolipoprotein B-100. But, of course you must remember that Lp(a) is just a form of LDL, and it too has apolipoprotein B-100 attached to it. So how would you know if you were really finding LDL within a plaque, and not Lp(a)? There is only one way to tell, really. See if you can find apolipoprotein(a) within plaques. If you can, it can only have come from Lp(a), not LDL.

Dr Rath decided to look for apolipoprotein(a) in areas of plaque formation, along with a team of other researchers, and they published their findings in the *European Heart Journal*. And guess what they found? That's right, a high concentration of apolipoprotein(a) within atherosclerotic plaques.

And Dr Rath is not the only one to find apolipoprotein(a) in plaques. A paper published in *Nature* in 1989 found exactly the same thing. In their words, which I will simplify afterwards:

We report here that apolipoprotein(a) interferes with endothelial cell fibrinolysis by inhibiting plasminogen binding and hence plasmin generation. In addition, we demonstrate lipoprotein(a) accumulation in atherosclerotic lesions. These findings may provide a link between impaired cell surface fibrinolysis and progressive atherosclerosis.

In short, this team also found apolipoprotein(a) in atherosclerotic plaques. They also confirmed that apolipoprotein(a) inhibits both the binding, and activity, of plasminogen within a blood clot.

This is fascinating research, but it is also research that is frowned upon by the powers that be. 'As we already know what causes heart disease, what exactly – young man – is the point of the research you are proposing? Grant application denied. And by the way, as a matter of interest, do you still enjoy working here?'

I hope it has become clear by now that Dr Matthias Rath is, in fact, a very clever chap. He worked out an entirely new hypothesis about heart disease. One that fits many of the known facts, and makes a lot more sense, frankly, than the LDL hypothesis. It's not difficult to see why Linus Pauling thought that Rath was on the right track. Personally, I think Rath has only a piece of the jigsaw puzzle in his hands. But it is a critically important piece.

My aim at this point, however, is not to delve too deeply into the Matthias Rath theory of heart disease. What I wanted to do was to give you enough information on an alternative view to accept that FH could cause heart disease, but not by raising LDL levels. And this is not just wild theorising – there is a lot of solid research behind it.

Indeed, once you start looking into this area, you find that FH is associated with a whole raft of other abnormalities, mostly to do with abnormal blood clotting. Just a couple of quick quotes on the matter from *Atherosclerosis* and the *British Haematology Journal* respectively:

> *The results suggest the hypercoagulability may play a role in the pathogenesis of coronary heart disease in patients with familial hypercholesterolaemia.*

> *Plasma fibrinogen [a clotting factor] was elevated in FH...*

In short, it is fully possible that FH causes an increase in the risk of heart disease, not by raising LDL levels, but through its impact on blood-clot formation.

However, I still think that the strongest argument against FH causing heart disease is that most people who die of heart disease do not have raised LDL levels. And most people with raised LDL levels do not die of heart disease, even people with FH. I think it is reasonable to ask, how can a raised LDL level be the cause of heart disease... when it is not present? And how can it be present and not cause heart disease? You're right, it can't.

HOW, EXACTLY, IS LDL SUPPOSED TO CAUSE HEART DISEASE?

Finally, in this chapter, I think it is reasonable to ask the question, 'If the establishment is so sure that LDL causes heart disease, how does it do it? What is the mechanism – where's the biological plausibility?' It's no good saying a thing causes heart disease then failing to provide a half-decent mechanism of action.

I think you should always bear in mind that the cholesterol hypothesis started life as the diet-heart hypothesis, with cholesterol in the diet as the major culprit substance. However, even Ancel Keys gave up on cholesterol in the diet pretty quickly. And, although saturated fat clings on in most people's minds, I hope you are convinced by now that it has no role. Which means that the first half of the hypothesis is dead.

But never mind, even with its legs cut off, researchers were still left with the 'fact' that raised cholesterol levels caused heart disease. Although what, exactly, is supposed to raise the cholesterol levels now is not clear. Even if were clear, it still can't be cholesterol in the blood that causes heart disease, because you don't have any cholesterol floating free in the blood.

Indeed, it was only quite late on that cholesterol was gently swept under the carpet, and LDL was introduced as the killer lipoprotein. At which point, presumably, people must have asked themselves something along the lines of: 'Finally we know what causes heart disease – it's LDL. But how does it do it?'

No one seems to have questioned how it can be that a hypothesis can go through several major changes, yet still somehow manage to remain the correct answer. All everyone wanted to do, it seems, was to hammer cholesterol into the jigsaw puzzle in some way – even if it had transformed itself into LDL along the way.

Personally, I would have more faith if the hypothesis had started life the right way round. The present thinking reminds me of the story of Keppler, who was determined to understand the orbits of planets around the sun. In his time it was decreed by the great thinkers that the planetary orbits had to fit within the 'perfect shapes' of the Greeks. For example, a perfect circle. Why did everyone think this? Because it had been decreed so by the Greeks, and they were all-knowing, and right about everything. You could not even dream of questioning their ancient Mumu wisdom.

Somewhat hampered by the requirement to get the facts to agree with the already-known answer, Keppler battled for 20 years to fit the observations of the 16th-century astronomer Tyco Brahe within the Greek ideal of perfect shapes. Unsurprisingly, he failed. Finally, Keppler gave up on the Greek idea of perfection, and thus were born Keppler's laws of planetary motion. Simultaneously, at least one section of the ancient wisdom of the Greeks was exposed for what it was – ridiculous dogmatic twaddle. You mean wise men in flowing gowns with beards aren't always right? Surely not.

Despite my philosophical objections, you may still think that everything had been sorted out by now, and that scientists with electron microscopes had watched LDL sticking to artery walls, or battling bravely through artery walls and then building up into a big plaque. Or something of the sort. The reality, however, is that researchers are still trying to work out how LDL creates atherosclerosis. It is true that huge tomes have been written on this subject outlining countless enzymes, and co-factors, and Lox-1 receptors and intracellular transportation systems. There is, literally, no end to it all. However, if it really is LDL that causes heart disease, I would like you to consider the following question. Why do we now hear so much about antioxidants? What's all that about? Why are they supposed to be so good for you? What have they got to do with LDL?

Well, you see, things have moved on a little. Now it is not actually LDL that's damaging, it is 'oxidised' LDL. Oxidised LDL is LDL that has reacted with oxygen, and can be thought of as slightly 'damaged'. A bit like leaving out meat uncovered overnight. Oxygen gets at it, reacts with it, and turns it into nasty wrinkly stuff. Of course, raised LDL is still important, but you must focus on oxidised LDL at the same time. Yet when you do you will find that it has miraculously changed shape back to LDL again. This area is a bit like quantum physics. The moment you focus on LDL it flips into oxidised LDL, and then when your attention slips, it flips back again. It is a veritable will o' the wisp that will never fully take form in front of you.

Indeed, if you ever start reading about this area you may find yourself filled with a desire to scream. 'Well, is it LDL, or oxidised LDL, will you make up your damned mind?' No chance: in general, those who write papers in this area give the impression that it is – sort of – both. By taking two positions simultaneously, this negates the tiresome requirement of formulating a hypothesis that can actually be disproved. You can keep on leaping backwards and forwards from one hypothesis to the other. I will simply make the general point that the 'oxidised' LDL hypothesis was primarily developed to explain how people with low LDL levels can get heart disease – while still claiming that LDL has a key role in the process. It's the old 'low is high' concept again.

Despite the fact that you cannot really get a handle on the 'oxidised LDL hypothesis', I think it does need some further explanation. However, I am not going to delve into this area in any great depth as it rapidly becomes incomprehensible.

To keep things as simple as possible then, the oxidised LDL hypothesis goes something like this (depending on which version you read). Endothelial cells posses a greater number of receptors for 'oxidised' LDL than receptors for normal LDL. This harmful, damaged, oxidised LDL is removed from the circulation by locking on to Lox-1 receptors on the surface endothelial cells. The oxidised LDL is then drawn into endothelial cell, transported through it, then ejected into the artery wall behind – although why an endothelial cell would want to do this is not clear. (And how an endothelial cell might do this is even more opaque.) After all, the liver has millions of receptors for oxidised LDL (Lox-1 receptors), and it sucks oxidised LDL from the circulation almost instantly – which is why there is very little oxidised LDL in the bloodstream: the liver doesn't like damaged goods in the blood. But if there is very little oxidised LDL in the bloodstream, then how... I know, I'm not going there.

Ignoring the fact that no one knows why endothelial cells would choose to eject oxidised LDL into the arterial wall behind it – or even how they do it – the theory states that once oxidised LDL starts to build up in the artery wall, white blood cells, called monocyctes, are attracted to the area to clear up the 'damaged' LDL. These monocytes then travel between the endothelial cells (converting themselves into macrophages) and set about absorbing the oxidised LDL and then… Well, they absorb so much oxidised LDL that they explode, as they have no off-switch to tell them that they have absorbed too much. No, I am not making this up. (OK, the technical term is 'rupture', but 'explode' sounds much more fun.)

Soon, more monocytes are attracted to the area. They too convert into macrophages, then over-fill to the point where they explode, and you are left with a big mass of dead macrophages, bits of oxidised LDL and lots of cholesterol, all floating about in a blob of goo. And that, ladies and gentlemen, is how an atherosclerotic plaque forms.

One question that no one seems to bother answering is this: how could such a process ever actually stop? If macrophages keep filling up and then exploding, we would seem to have a positive feedback loop on our hands. The more oxidised LDL there is, the more monocytes are attracted to the area, they convert into macrophages, gorge themselves to the point where they explode, releasing more oxidised goo. More monocytes are attracted, more explosions, more goo. This process does not appear to have any off switch. Or if there is, researchers are keeping remarkably quiet about it. It's just another one of the many fault lines in heart-disease research where people – rather than answering the question – start using high-speed jargon, change the subject, or say things like, 'Moving on, it is now clear that…'

Anyway, according to the oxidised LDL theory it is not the level of LDL that matters, it is the level of oxidised LDL in the bloodstream that is important. Thus, if you can find substances that act as antioxidants, e.g. vitamin E, beta-carotene and vitamin C – the sort of things found in green-leaf tea – you will stop LDL from getting oxidised and prevent heart disease. Frankly, if you believe this, you will believe anything.

I don't even need to believe it. Because no study on antioxidants has managed to unearth any difference, whatsoever, in the rate of heart disease between those taking the antioxidants and those taking the placebo. Of course, this has made no difference to anything at all.'It was the wrong sort of antioxidants, you see.' Don't worry, until a positive study appears (which is going to happen by chance at some point), it always will be the wrong sort of antioxidants. Then, suddenly, it will be just the right sort.

The oxidised LDL hypothesis is not the only new hypothesis to spring up in an attempt to shoehorn in LDL as the primary cause of heart disease. We now have not one but three mainstream competing hypotheses. This hardly suggests that things are heading towards a speedy resolution, with only a few loose ends to tidy up.

The simple fact of the matter is that after many decades, and hundreds of millions of pounds spent, no one truly has the faintest idea exactly how LDL causes heart disease. But you would never believe this from listening to the experts talk, and reading what they write. LDL still rules supreme.

Personally, I find it rather weird that as I listen to yet another opinion leader outlining complex discussions on LDL receptor down-regulation of this, and microtubular transcytosis system that, I too come to think that this has all been proven. Bullshit truly does baffle brains. Yes, now you put it like that… Yes… I can see the Emperor's clothes. They truly are magnificent. Thank God I am finally able to see what everyone else can see.

At times like this, I always try to pull myself back and think what question an intelligent child might ask about all of this. What are the 'stand-out' problems with the LDL hypothesis that just cannot be explained, no matter how hard you try? I think that there are three killer questions. And they are these:

- Why don't veins develop atherosclerosis?
- Why does atherosclerosis develop in discrete (separate) plaques?
- If a high LDL level causes atherosclerosis, how can people with low LDL levels get the same disease?

Why don't veins develop atherosclerosis?

You may think that veins and arteries are very different. However, in general structure, arteries and veins both have a thin inner lining, one cell thick, known as the endothelium. Behind this lies a thicker layer made up of muscle and connective tissue – known as the media. Wrapped around this, and holding the blood vessel together, is the externa.

In basic structure, therefore, arteries and veins are identical. Indeed, they start life exactly the same way in the embryo. The only difference is that arteries are thicker than veins because they have to deal with a higher blood pressure. You might think of a vein as a puny artery that has not done enough exercise. (Proof of this later.)

Given that fact that veins and arteries have exactly the same structure, and are exposed to exactly the same level of LDL, oxidised or otherwise, you would think, would you not, that if LDL causes plaques to develop in an artery it would also cause atherosclerotic plaques to develop in a vein? If it is a case of LDL somehow passing though the endothelium into the artery wall, and this is a function of the level of LDL in the blood. Yet atherosclerosis never develops in veins. Ponder that thought for a moment, and see if you can come up with an answer that involves LDL as a cause. Because I can't.

Actually, I have to admit that I haven't been entirely truthful here. If you take a vein from the leg and transplant it to the heart – as is done in a coronary artery bypass graft – the 'vein' rapidly develops severe atherosclerosis. Which means that veins can develop atherosclerosis, if you make them do the job of an artery. Perhaps of even greater interest is that one group of researchers did the reverse to a bypass graft: they took a bit of an artery and grafted it into a vein. OK, they did in rabbits, not humans, but I still think it is enlightening to see what happened:

> *Three months after surgery, grafted arteries possess similar structures as that of veins. The artery interposed to vein did not develop atherosclerosis and underwent atrophic remodeling.*

Effectively – in rabbits, at least – if you insert a bit of artery into a vein, the artery wall narrows and thins until you are left with something that looks identical to a vein – in fact, it is a vein. Not only that, the converted artery/vein is immune to developing atherosclerosis.

What does this prove? Well, think about it logically:

- Veins and arteries are exposed to identical levels of LDL.
- Arteries develop atherosclerosis.
- Veins don't.
- Replace an artery with a vein, and the vein develops atherosclerosis.
- Replace a vein with an artery, and the artery is protected against atherosclerosis.

Conclusion: something about the position of arteries within the body or the job they do causes atherosclerosis to develop. That something cannot be LDL, or oxidised LDL, because this factor remains constant throughout the circulatory system.

Why does atherosclerosis develop in discrete plaques?
Another major problem with the LDL hypothesis is the fact that, even in severely diseased individuals, most arterial walls are completely unaffected. If the level of LDL, oxidised or otherwise, is the main cause, how come some bits of artery don't get touched?

To my mind, if raised LDL causes atherosclerosis through some form of excess exposure, then finding discrete patches of atherosclerosis is akin to lying in the sun all day, yet only getting sunburned in a few small patches, the rest of the skin remaining unaffected. How likely does this seem? Not very, I would suggest.

This, I suppose, is actually a similar problem to the vein/artery conundrum. Why don't veins get atherosclerosis, and why are some areas of arteries vulnerable, while others are not? If LDL is leaking through the endothelium, or being transported through endothelium (or whatever is supposed to be happening), and then entering the arterial wall behind, this should happen everywhere, in all arteries. Unless… some bits of the arterial tree – e.g. coronary arteries, carotid arteries, or bits where blood flow changes direction quickly – are exposed to greater flow turbulence, and this causes damage to these areas, so plaques form at these places. If you are thinking this, then I would agree with you.

But what you would probably then go on to ponder is that plaques start at areas of endothelial damage – fine, no problem with that – but LDL does not damage the endothelium, no matter what the level. What damages the endothelium therefore, has to be something else. Ergo, something else causes heart disease.

If a high LDL level causes atherosclerosis, how can people with low LDL levels get the same disease?

Now to look at my final problem. How can high levels of cholesterol cause heart disease if people with low levels get exactly the same disease? This would be the only example in recorded history of a factor causing a disease when it isn't even there.

There are two mainstream ad-hoc hypotheses designed to deal with this problem. The first is to claim that it is oxidised LDL that is the problem – see above for my response to this incoherent ad-hoc hypothesis thingy. The second is to claim that no one in the West has a low LDL level – that we all have high levels. Yes, every single one of us. Ho-hum, here we go again.

I have to admit, though, that the 'everyone in the West has a high cholesterol level' argument is a cracker. It's complete rubbish, of course, but it carries a kind of eerie power. Primarily because 'everyone in the West', it seems to me, is truly convinced that we have all fallen from the higher state of grace granted to primitive people who are 'at one' with nature. We listen not to the great goddess Gaia as we plunder the world of its riches, isolated in our metal carapaces (cars), disconnected from the ebb and flow of the seasons and nature itself. Numb to the wondrous circle of life. Yes, I know, I feel terribly guilty too. But I can still comfort myself, just a little, with my vastly improved life expectancy, freedom from nasty infections and infestations, Bose hi-fi system, air-con in the car and suchlike. The occasional malt whisky also helps.

The high priest of the 'primitive is best' philosophy is Dr JH O'Keefe Jr. This, from a recent paper produced by Dr O'Keefe along with four of his colleagues:

Optimal low-density lipoprotein is 50 to 70 mg/dl:
lower is better and physiologically normal
*The normal low-density lipoprotein (LDL) cholesterol range is 50
to 70 mg/dl for native hunter-gatherers, healthy human
neonates, free-living primates, and other wild mammals (all of
whom do not develop atherosclerosis). Randomized trial data
suggest atherosclerosis progression and coronary heart disease
events are minimized when LDL is lowered to <70 mg/dl. No
major safety concerns have surfaced in studies that lowered LDL
to this range of 50 to 70 mg/dl. The current guidelines setting the
target LDL at 100 to 115 mg/dl may lead to substantial
undertreatment in high-risk individuals.*

By the way, 50–70mg/dl in US units converts to 1.3–1.8mmol/l in UK units. This is considerably less than half the current average LDL level in the UK. For the vast majority of us, the only way you could get your LDL level this low would be to take a high-dose statin for the rest of your life. Based on current figures, this would mean 99 per cent of the population of the western world taking statins – forever. On that basis, I make Pfizer a buy.

Perhaps, at this point, it would be tempting to name other names and outline how much money is spent on first-class flights, slap-up dinners etc by the statin manufacturers . Indeed, I would like to, but my publisher say's it is too hazardous. Of course disclosure of doctors' links to pharmaceutical companies is freely available if you care to look.

Indeed you would surely find it easier to pass through the eye of a needle than to find an eminent cardiologist who has not been paid... (Sorry, they are not paid, they are given honoraria. Start again.) You can hardly find an eminent cardiologist who has not been given honoraria by at least one pharmaceutical company that manufactures statins. And the sums involved are far from small. We are talking, in many cases, hundreds of thousands of dollars per year. I know, for I – ahem – have signed some of the cheques.

By way of illustrating the connections between industry and opinion leaders, it might be interesting to look at the American National Cholesterol Education Program (NCEP). This is a hugely influential body in the USA that has developed three sets of guidelines on LDL lowering, each time revising their treatment level for LDL further downwards. Where they lead, all others follow.

The last set of NCEP guidelines actually caused a bit of an outcry. Here is a section of an article that appeared in the *Washington Post* at the time:

> On July 13, the National Cholesterol Education Program (NCEP), part of the National Institutes of Health, unveiled tougher guidelines for cholesterol levels – guidelines so stringent that millions of Americans at risk of heart disease would have to take costly statin drugs to meet the new lower limits. What the NCEP didn't unveil was that most panel members who helped write the recommendations had financial ties to the pharmaceutical companies that stood to gain enormously from increased use of statins.
>
> Critics immediately complained about the hidden financial ties, and demanded disclosure. Within days, the highly respected sponsors of the cholesterol guidelines – the NIH, the American Heart Association (AHA) and the American College of Cardiology (ACC) – posted the disclosures on the NCEP's web site. The extent of the connections was stunning: of the nine members of the panel that wrote the guidelines, six had each received research grants, speaking honoraria or consulting fees from at least three and in some cases all five of the manufacturers of statins; only one had no financial links at all.
>
> If all the members with conflicts had recused themselves, in fact, only two would have been left.
>
> That didn't look too good, so a day or so later, another note

*appeared on the site, attempting to make the guidelines seem
more credible. It explained that the panel's draft proposals had
been 'subjected to multiple layers of scientific review,' first by the
NCEP's coordinating committee, 'consisting of 35 representatives
of leading medical, public health, voluntary, community, and
citizen organizations and Federal agencies,' and then by the
scientific and steering committees of the heart association and
the college of cardiology. 'Altogether approximately 90 reviewers
scrutinized the draft,' the note said. So the message to the public:
No need to worry about pro-industry bias.'*

Jerome Kassirer [Editor in Chief emeritus of the
New England Journal of Medicine *and a professor
at the Tufts University School of Medicine.]*

Actually, there was another bit of this article that I really enjoyed. It was
part of a discussion about how bias can creep into collective decisions:
'*When companies with identical interests are underwriting virtually all the
researchers, decision makers can become susceptible to "group think." The
military has a name for this sort of trap – "incestuous amplification."*'

I love the concept of incestuous amplification. Never was a truer
phrase coined than this. I knew that there had to be some
psychological explanation for the collective madness surrounding LDL
levels and treatment with statins. My phrase for it was the 'tyranny of
conformity'. But I prefer 'incestuous amplification'. It sounds much more
pathological and in need of treatment.

This all concerns me greatly. These guidlines carry real weight with
the medical proffession and the public and it is therefore essential that
the public have confidence in the process that produces them. Where
else in an area of critical endeavour would such a potential conflict of
interest be allowed?

Anyway, to return to the main point, which is the ad-hoc hypothesis
that 'everyone in the West has a high cholesterol level'. I shall just run
through the argument again. In comparison to 'primitive man', everyone
in the West has a cholesterol level that is far too high. Thus, everyone in

the West who dies of heart disease automatically must have have a high cholesterol level.' Huzzah! You've got to admit, this knocks teleoanalysis into a cocked hat. Everyone is abnormal, and all shall be treated.

But how can this argument actually be supported? We have no idea what the 'healthy' cholesterol levels of our free-range ancestors might have been – surely we must be guessing? Not so. You see, according to JH O'Keefe Jr, we should look at the surviving communities of hunter-gatherers left in the world, animals in the wild, and infants as yet 'uncontaminated' by a western lifestyle. By analysing these groups, we should be able to see what a natural, healthy, 'primitive' LDL level should be – the level that we should strive to attain. In his words:

> The normal low-density lipoprotein (LDL) cholesterol range is 50 to 70 mg/dl [1.3–1.8mmol/l] for native hunter-gatherers, healthy human neonates, free-living primates, and other wild mammals (all of whom do not develop atherosclerosis).

While on the surface this sounds sort of reasonable, in reality it is complete balls. Let's just open up this statement a little bit more. Firstly, I would like to point out that a healthy human neonate is a child under the age of four weeks. What can their LDL level tell us about healthy adult levels? Precisely nothing.

Would O'Keefe like to argue that neonatal blood pressure also represents the 'ideal' for adult blood pressure? The average blood pressure of a neonate is about 80/40. If you found that level in an adult it would indicate massive blood loss, shock and imminent death. So maybe it's not that healthy after all. In fact, maybe healthy neonates are just a smidge different to healthy adults, and the two should not really be compared.

Moving on to the free-living primates, and other wild animals. The animals he chose were:

- Baboon
- Howler monkey

- Night monkey
- Horse
- Boar
- Peccary
- Black rhinoceros
- African elephant

I know that at this point you must think I am starting to make this up. Oh gracious me, no. I have spent many an evening amusing myself by reading his paper. It ranks right up there with teleoanalysis in my pantheon of great medical papers with which you can use to light your barbecue. If you want to read the full version merely type in the following web address:
http://www.thepaleodiet.com/articles/JACC%20LDL%20Final.pdf

I thought it might be interesting to match the cholesterol levels, and life expectancy, of the animals O'Keefe chose against those of humans:

Boar: Cholesterol level 1.5mmol/l – life expectancy 4–5 years
Baboon: Cholesterol level 2.1mmol/l – life expectancy 30 years
Adult American: Cholesterol level 5.8mmol/l – life expectancy 72 years

Frankly, I gave up at that point. Mainly because I thought that using the cholesterol levels of other species to make a point about human health was utter and complete... words fail me... the world is going dark. Rosebud... rosebud....

Where was I? Oh yes, the hummingbird, for example, has a 'healthy' blood-sugar level that is five times that of humans. So what? So absolutely nothing at all. A full-grown bull African elephant weighs about six tons. Is that a healthy weight for a human being?

Perhaps you feel that it is still useful to look at the hunter-gatherer communities that O'Keefe chose. They were: the Hazda, the Inuit, the IKung, the Pygmy and the San. Average cholesterol levels were about

2.7mmol/l among these five groups. And yes, it's true, they also had a very low rate of heart disease.

But I thought it might also be educational to look at the reported life expectancy of these five groups:

San   = 36 years
Hazda   = 32.5 years
IKung   = 30 years
Pygmy   = 17 years
Inuit   = 'Inuit have the lowest life expectancy of all Aboriginal peoples [in Canada], followed by those living on-reserve.' [I couldn't get an accurate figure, I think it's about 55 years.]

Should we really aspire to reach their super-low cholesterol levels? If we did, could we also look forward to achieving their super-low life expectancy? You think these things are unconnected? Iribarren would argue strongly that very low cholesterol levels are a sign of serious underlying illness, which is why people in the West with low cholesterol levels have such a terrible life expectancy. (By the way, of course hunter-gatherers have very low rates of heart disease – before they reach the age at which heart disease is likely to strike, they are already dead.)

I believe we should ignore extreme examples of horribly unhealthy populations with terrible life expectancies, and look instead at healthy populations with a long life expectancy, e.g. those in North America, Japan and all countries in western Europe. Here, it is blindingly clear that a cholesterol level of 2.7mmol/l is neither normal, nor optimal. It is a sign of ill health and imminent death.

When cholesterol levels in Japan rose from an unhealthy 3.9mmol/l to a much more 'normal' and healthy 4.9 mmol/l, life expectancy increased, and death from all forms of cardiovascular disease fell dramatically. But hey, if you prefer to support your argument by analysing the cholesterol levels of two-week-old children, baboons, black rhinoceroses, elephants, the IKung and the Hazda, that is entirely up to you.

In reality, using the 'totality of the evidence', it seems clear that a cholesterol level between something like 5.0mmol/l and 6.5mmol/l is normal for healthy adult humans, as it is associated with the greatest life expectancy. On this basis, something around 5.5–6.0mmol/l is average.

And if we use the figure of about 5.7mmol/l as bang-on average, the facts would say that approximately 50 per cent of people who die of heart disease have high cholesterol levels and 50 per cent are below average. Which removes cholesterol as a risk factor entirely.

The Framingham risk score

Just before signing off on this section, I thought I should mention something else: the 'Framingham risk score'. This has been developed over the years using the major risk factors discovered in the population of Framingham, near Boston, to calculate your risk of dying of heart disease.

To look at this scoring system, you would get the impression that absolutely everything about risk of heart disease had been worked out to the nearest fraction of a percentage point. There is nothing left to discover. Plug yourself into the Framingham risk calculator and you can work out your risk to within a 1 per cent tolerance. To do this, you use the following criteria:

- Sex (gender)
- Age
- Total cholesterol levels
- Smoking status
- HDL level
- Blood pressure (systolic)

(Some tables also add in whether or not you are diabetic.)

Each of the above criteria has points attached, e.g. if you are a man aged between 20–34, this age gives you a score of -9. If you are a man aged between 50–54, this age gives you a score of +6. If you are a man aged between 50–54 and you have a cholesterol level between

5.0mmol/l and 5.5mmol/l, your cholesterol level at this age scores an additional 4 points – and so on.

Once you have added up all your points, you then reference the handy percentage risk ready-reckoner. Then you find, just to give a couple of examples, that a fifteen-point total equates to a three per cent risk of developing heart disease over the next ten years. Nineteen points equates to a ten-year risk of eight per cent.

This is all incredibly precise – is it not? Well, if you are a white, Protestant, American male living near Boston, it is. But what about other populations? A study in Italy used the Framingham risk score and found that:

> *The estimated number of coronary events by the Framingham function was 2,425 in women while that observed was only 1,181 (ratio 2.1). In men 9,919 events were expected and only 3,706 were observed (ratio 2.7).*

In short, if you want to make the male Framingham risk score work in Italy, you have to divide by 2.7. If you want to make the Framingham risk score work in France, you actually need to divide by 4. So we have this fantastically accurate calculator of cardiovascular risk, which overestimates risk in Italy by 2.7 and in France by 4.

Even in the UK, which is much more like the US in overall heart-disease risk, the Framingham risk data was hardly accurate.

> *When the Framingham Risk Equation using cholesterol levels was applied to British men for ten years, it was found that 84% of the heart disease occurred in the men classified as low risk!*
> *Furthermore, 75% of the men classified as high risk using the Framingham Risk data were still free of heart disease ten years later. It seems the equation is still missing a few important variables.*
> BMJ, 29 November 2003; 327(7426): 1267.

Looking in the other direction, if you apply the Framingham risk calculator to Australian Aboriginals it is capable of underestimating the risk by up to thirtyfold:

> *The observed incidence was about four and three times the predicted incidence for age groups <35 and 35–44 years, respectively, and about twice the predicted incidence for those over 45 years of age. The Framingham function was a particularly unreliable predictor for women, especially younger women, in whom the observed CHD rate was* **30 times the predicted rate** *[my emphasis].*
> *http://www.mja.com.au/public/issues/182_02_170105/wan10439_fm.html*

In summary: if you use the Framingham risk score for French men, it overestimates risk by 400 per cent. If you use it for younger Australian Aboriginal women, it can underestimate the risk by 3,000 per cent. Which gives a tolerance of 12,000 per cent. Let's put it this way: I hope the people who developed the Framingham risk score aren't designing aeroplanes. At least, not any aeroplane that I am going to fly on.

However, my main takeaway point from this is the following. The Framingham risk score, with its exact measurements, and exact calculations, gives the very strong impression that the mainstream research community now knows all the risk factors for heart disease in exact detail, fully understands them, and can control them. Everything important has been discovered. And if you were to follow the advice of the experts you could probably avoid heart disease altogether. The reality, however, is that almost nothing is explained by the conventional risk factors. If an Australian Aboriginal man can have exactly the same risk factors as a French man, and yet have 16 times the rate of heart disease, this means that the conventional risk factors can only explain a maximum of 6.25 per cent of the total risk of heart disease, which leaves another 93.75 per cent lurking out there, yet to be discovered.

The high priests of heart disease may wish to give the impression that they have the required wisdom to keep death at bay. The reality is that they haven't got a clue. You might as well resort to blood sacrifices and drilling holes in the side of your head. Did someone call for leeches?

CHAPTER 8

STATINS AND HEART DISEASE

'Statins lower the LDL level and protect against heart disease.' This is the only fact that really matters; all else is so much hot air, do I hear you say? On the face of it, the data certainly seems to represent the so-called 'reversibility of effect', which is considered one of the strongest forms of scientific proof – for good reason.

If you think factor x causes disease y, then you remove factor x and disease y disappears. 'Well... HOW MUCH MORE PROOF DO YOU WANT?' A bit more, actually. Firstly, with statins, even if you get the LDL level down to about 2mmol/l, you reduce the relative risk of dying of heart disease by about 30 per cent, absolute max. Which means that you can completely remove the risk factor – high LDL levels – yet people still die of heart disease.

Statin data are one thing. The interpretation and presentation of data on statins is another. Here, for example, is a press release from the British Heart Foundation about the Heart Protection Study, published in 2004 – the last really big statin study to report:

> *Heart experts call for urgent action to implement new findings*
> *on cholesterol-lowering treatment*
> *Tens of thousands of lives could be saved each year by changing*
> *prescribing guidelines for statins, say UK researchers*

Research reported in tomorrow's [Saturday 6 July] Lancet is set to revolutionise the way cholesterol-lowering drugs are prescribed. It shows that using 'statin' drugs to lower blood cholesterol levels protects a far wider range of people at risk of heart attacks and strokes than had previously been thought to benefit. These findings should lead to major changes in treatment guidelines, preventing tens of thousands of deaths each year, a London news briefing has been told.

*At present, statins are often restricted to people who have heart disease and elevated cholesterol levels. But, new findings from the UK's 20,000-patient Heart Protection Study show that statins also cut the risks of heart attacks and strokes in people who have diabetes, or have narrowing of arteries in their legs, or have had a stroke. **Most remarkably, the study found substantial benefits even among those high-risk patients considered to have 'normal' or 'low' cholesterol levels. It provides definite evidence that guidelines should be changed so that – irrespective of the blood cholesterol level – a statin is considered for anybody at increased risk of either heart attacks or strokes.***

'The clear message from this study is: "Treat risk – not cholesterol level'," said Professor Sir Charles George, Medical Director of the British Heart Foundation – the UK's leading heart charity. He called for an urgent review of national and international guidelines on statin use by government organisations, such as the National Institute of Clinical Excellence (NICE) in the UK and the National Institutes of Health (NIH) in the USA, as well as by professional bodies, such as the European Society of Cardiology (ESC) and the American Heart Association (AHA).

The study overturns conventional wisdom in a number of other areas. For example, current guidelines say that there is little evidence that statins help older individuals. By deliberately studying large numbers of older people, the researchers were able to show that cholesterol-lowering with

statins was just as effective for the over 70s as for those in middle age.

Likewise, not many women had been included in previous studies so there was little direct evidence on the benefits and safety of statins in women. With more than 5,000 women included in the Heart Protection Study, it has been able to show that statins work just as well for women as for men.

HPS lead investigator Professor Rory Collins said: 'HPS shows unequivocally that statins can produce substantial benefit in a very much wider range of high-risk people than had been thought. These new findings are relevant to the treatment of some hundreds of millions of people worldwide. If now, as a result, an extra 10 million high-risk people were to go onto statin treatment, this would save about 50,000 lives a year – that's a thousand each week. In addition, this would prevent similar numbers of people from suffering non-fatal heart attacks or strokes.

The HPS team estimates that implementing these new findings fully would more than triple the numbers of people benefiting from statins. In the UK, the numbers treated with statins would increase from a current figure of less than 1 in 20 of the population aged over 40 (or about 1 million people) to about 1 in 8 (about 3 million people). This would save an extra 10,000 lives each year.

Yee-haaa! How fantastic is that, we can save tens of thousands of lives by prescribing a few million more statins a day. A thousand lives a week in the UK alone! And this gushing praise does not come from a paid PR agency in full bullshit mode. It comes from ultra-respectable sources. *The Lancet*, Oxford University, Professor Sir Charles George, Medical Director of the British Heart Foundation no less. If you could win an argument by the sheer number of gongs and letters after your name, I would have been beaten into a senseless mush by now, a white towel fluttering despondently on to the canvas.

However I hope that, by now, you may recognise that, despite the glow of eminence, this press release is actually riven with gaping holes.

Here are a few statements that are worth a bit more analysis:

'It [the study] provides definite evidence that guidelines should be changed so that – irrespective of the blood cholesterol level *[my emphasis]* – *a statin is considered for anybody at increased risk of either heart attacks or strokes.*

So we should be treating everyone at risk of heart disease with statins, no matter what their cholesterol level. Why? Because statins reduce the risk at all cholesterol levels. High, average, or low. Just ponder that statement for a moment or two. Do you find anything strange about it?

While you do that. Here's another statement:

By deliberately studying large numbers of older people, the researchers were able to show that cholesterol-lowering with statins was just as effective for the over 70s as for those in middle age.

But a high cholesterol level is not a risk factor in the over 70s. If anything, raised cholesterol protects against heart disease in the over 70s, especially in women – for whom, in fact, a raised cholesterol level isn't a risk factor for heart disease at any age.

Another of the main findings of the HPS was that it protected against stroke – much more so than against heart disease. Yet, a raised cholesterol level is NOT a risk factor for stroke. Probably the exact opposite, if truth be told.

Were any of these issues raised, or even hinted at? In the press release? Not at all. Statins are marvellous, everyone should take them, end of discussion.

However, the issues I have just raised are as trifles compared to the elephant that is sitting in the middle of the room here. It sits quietly cleaning its tusks, unremarked upon, but it is there nonetheless, no matter how much mainstream researchers would like it to pack up its trunk and trumpety, trump, trump, off to the circus. This elephant even has a name. It is called 'Nellie the total mortality data'. Not a very snappy name, I agree, but it is fully accurate.

STATINS AND TOTAL MORTALITY

With more than 5,000 women included in the Heart Protection Study, it has been able to show that statins work just as well for women as for men.

That rather depends on what you mean by *work*, I suppose. What I mean by work is that statins saved lives. The HPS team, however, decided not to release the total mortality data on women.

I was not the only one to notice this. Arnold Jenkins, a UK GP, picked up on this not insignificant point, and wrote about it in the *BMJ*:

Imagine my delight when I heard of the large heart protection study showing clear benefits in the use of statins for women. On reading this study I was therefore disappointed to find the total mortality data for women missing. I now understand that the total mortality benefit for women did not reach significance and therefore was not published.

Louise Bowman, personal communication, 2002
http://bmj.bmjjournals.com/cgi/content/full/327/7420/933-b

I too, have attempted to get hold of the mortality data for women from the HPS study. No such luck. Overall mortality is the most important end point in any clinical trial. It is also the easiest to measure. The HPS researchers are not actually alone in failing to publish overall mortality data in women. This is also true of most of the statin trials, although on those occasions when it has been published, it has shown nothing at all. The 4S, one of the earliest, and by far the most positive of all the statin trials ever, showed no difference at all in female mortality. (Actually, two more women in the trial who were taking statins died, but this was a 'non-significant' difference.) In short, statins do not save lives in women.

Statins do not save lives in women.

Statins do not save lives in women.

Statins do not save lives in women.

Is it possible to highlight how important this fact actually is?

STATINS DO NOT SAVE LIVES IN WOMEN!

But you would never know that from reading anything that is written on the subject. You have to dig and dig. This information is buried very deeply. Actually, that is not quite true. The information isn't buried, it just plain doesn't exist. And how can you find something that doesn't exist?

Firstly, you have to ask yourself the most difficult question of all: 'What's missing?' It's a bit like 'the dog that didn't bark'. It's not what happened that's important, it's what didn't happen. While our attention is distracted by 50,000 lives being saved from heart disease every year, we fail to spot the total mortality data escaping through a hole in the floor.

As a man, I can't truly speak for women. But ladies, I really think that you should be outraged by the complete silence on this issue. When your doctor is badgering you to take a statin, do you not think that it might be of some importance for them to mention that, while this pill may slightly reduce your risk of stroke and heart disease, it will not on average increase your life expectancy by one single day? Or, to put it another way, taking a statin may change what is written on your death certificate, but it will not change the date.

Despite the complete and utter lack of evidence of any mortality benefit, GPs in the UK are actively encouraged to check cholesterol levels in women, and further encouraged to get the cholesterol level below 5.0mmol/l. If they achieve this in a high enough percentage of their practice population, they are then paid large sums of money.

If this were not so serious it would be laughable. But frankly, at this point, I do not feel like laughing. I feel like grabbing a few people by the lapels and shaking them with great vigour. How can you justify putting millions upon millions of women on powerful and potentially very damaging drugs, when they will not save one single life? This question requires an answer.

If this book achieves nothing else but to start a debate on this issue, then I will be perfectly content – as it is a debate that can have only one conclusion. Perhaps you think statins are harmless, so it doesn't really matter all that much? Well, if you are a foetus, statins are not harmless at all.

While it is certainly true that not many women of childbearing age take statins, it is becoming more and more common. And with statins now available over the counter in the UK, there is an increasing danger that warnings about taking statins in pregnancy will go unheeded. Or perhaps someone will forget to mention it as they hand over a pack of statins on a busy afternoon in the supermarket pharmacy. Or maybe a husband will pick them up for his wife, without telling anyone that they are not for him.

I have been told that this can't possibly happen, because statins are contraindicated in pregnancy. Well, so are about ten thousand other drugs, most of which have never actually been shown to do harm. If a drug hasn't been tested in pregnant women – and which company would now risk doing this – it is often 'contraindicated', just to be on the safe side.

However, there are degrees of contraindication. Roaccutane, for example is hyper-contraindicated. This drug is used for resistant acne, and can only be prescribed by a dermatologist with severe warnings handed out about getting pregnant, and instant termination recommended if this happens. Why? Because of the terrible birth defects that this drug can cause.

Roaccutane represents a full-on contraindication, one that is taken very seriously indeed. This is a long way from the 'It's probably not a good idea, but it probably won't do any harm' type of contraindication. Or the contraindication against certain forms of antibiotic because they can cause permanent tooth discolouration – which is unfortunate, but hardly life threatening.

In short, to say that a drug is 'contraindicated' in pregnancy does not necessarily ring many alarm bells. And where, in doctor's minds, do statins sit on this spectrum of contraindication? Pretty low down, to judge by my discussions with fellow doctors.

Making things even more likely to go wrong, statins have been presented as a universal panacea, with no side effects worth mentioning. Taking a statin is now viewed, among doctors, as akin to taking a multivitamin or low-dose aspirin.

You may remember a quote from Dr John Reckless about the use of statins:

> *So maybe people should be able to have their statin, perhaps if not in their drinking water, with their drinking water.*

Statins can now be bought in the UK without a prescription. In this climate women will take statins over the counter, and will become pregnant while on statins. This is inevitable – it has almost certainly already happened.

But be afraid, be very afraid. In April 2004 an article appeared in the *New England Journal of Medicine* entitled 'Central nervous system and limb anomalies in case reports of first-trimester statin exposure'. As statins are 'contraindicated' in pregnancy, there wasn't much data to go on. But they still managed to find 178 cases. This number was whittled down through first-trimester elective and spontaneous abortions, loss to follow-up, and suchlike, to an eventual figure of 52 confirmed cases.

Out of these 52 there were 20 reports of malformation, including severe defects of the nervous system, unilateral limb deficiencies, complex lower-limb abnormalities and much more.

Here are just three of the reports:

- Holoprosencephly (defective septum separating lateral cerebral ventricles, with cerebral dysfunction), atrial septal defect, aortic hypoplasia, death at one month of age.
- Cervicothoracic-to-lumbar neural tube defect, myelocele, duplication of spinal cord, cerebellar herniation with hydrocephalus; apparent agenesis of palate.
- Left leg: femur 16% shorter than right side; foot: aplasia of metatarsals and phalanges 3,4 and 5; additional VACTERL

defects[8]: left renal dysplasia reversed laterality of aorta, disorganised lumbosacral vertebrae, single umbilical artery; additional findings: clitoral hypertrophy, vaginal and uterine agenesis.

As the authors point out, data from case series cannot be used to test hypotheses of teratogenicity (substances causing birth defects). But 20 severe birth defects out of 52 children is an extremely disturbing figure. As high as anything found with thalidomide, and with more serious defects.

I believe this study constitutes proof that statins are extremely dangerous in pregnancy, and cause terrible birth defects, a belief that is reinforced by the fact that the defects fit within the known effects of inhibiting cholesterol synthesis in the foetus. Oh yes, statins are truly wonder drugs. We should be putting them into the water supply. Just don't expect too many healthy babies to emerge if we do. A few hundred thousand with 'duplication of the spinal cord', perhaps.

Before getting pulled down too far into the damaging effects of statins – an issue that I will return to – I want to get back to the overall mortality data. This time in men.

TOTAL MORTALITY IN MEN

At this point in the discussion I need to split men into two distinct types:

Type A: Those who already have diagnosed heart disease (previous heart attack, or angina).
Type B: Those who don't.

This distinction has become blurred more recently – I would say quite deliberately – into high risk and low risk. However, it is a very important distinction to make. Because, according to the clinical trials, if you give statins to men who already have heart disease they are protected

8 VACTERL association means finding three or more of the following: vertebral, anal, cardiac, tracheal, oesophageal, renal and limb defects.

against cardiovascular disease. They also have a reduced overall mortality rate (more on this later).

However, if you give statins to men who do not have heart disease, while you do reduce the rate of cardiovascular disease, there is no benefit on overall mortality. None at all. And you don't need to take my word for it.

The University of British Columbia, which is part of the worldwide Cochrane collaboration – a not-for-profit group that analyses health-care interventions around the world – decided to look at the use of statins in primary prevention, that is, in people with no known pre-existing heart disease. (Secondary prevention is attempting to reduce death from CVD in people who already have heart disease.)

The researchers at the University of Columbia asked the question 'Do statins have a role in primary prevention?' And they brought together the data from the major statin studies done around the world. The answer:

- *If cardiovascular serious adverse events are viewed in isolation, 71 primary prevention patients with cardiovascular risk factors have to be treated with a statin for 3 to 5 years to prevent one myocardial infarction or stroke.*
- *This cardiovascular benefit is not reflected in two measures of overall health impact, total mortality and total serious adverse events. Therefore, statins have not been shown to provide an overall health benefit in primary prevention trials.*

Dr Graham Jackson, in the UK, also looked at all of the statin trials done up to the year 2000. His conclusion, published in the *British Journal of Clinical Pharmacology*, was that:

> *Long term use of statins for primary prevention of heart disease produced a 1% greater risk of death over ten years vs placebo when the result of all the big controlled trials reported before 2000 were combined.*

And that, ladies and gentlemen, is the bottom line. Statins do not reduce mortality in men who do not already have diagnosed heart disease, which represents considerably more than 90 per cent of the male population.

As a slight aside, after the publication of these data, someone asked the University of British Columbia researchers the question: 'What is the evidence of benefit for primary prevention in women, in heart disease?' Their reply:

> There were 10,990 women in the primary prevention trials (28% of the total). Only coronary events were reported for women, but when these were pooled they were not reduced by statin therapy... Thus the coronary benefit in primary prevention trials appears to be limited to men.

In short, in primary prevention, statins not only have zero effect on overall mortality, they also have zero effect on reducing heart disease in women. So you get absolutely no benefits at all. I suppose this may all seem almost unbelievable, given the ludicrous levels of hype surrounding statins, but it's true.

However, studies such as the one done by the University of British Columbia have been brushed aside by the statin juggernaut, with no discernible effect on anyone, or anything. If anything, the hype has merely accelerated. For example, a couple of years ago a major trial (ASCOT-LLA), was stopped early – an unusual step. The reason for this is because of the 'massive' reduction in cardiovascular deaths in those given statins, compared to those poor souls condemned to taking a placebo. The difference was so great even though the trial was blinded that it was considered unethical to continue.*

> *As the cardiovascular benefits in patients taking Lipitor were highly significant, the independent Steering Committee stopped*

---

* Clinical trials are usually 'blinded'. That is, neither the doctor nor the patient knows if they are getting the drug. However, some researchers have access to certain blinded data, to check up on whether or not too many deaths are occurring in the different patient groups for the trial to continue.

the cholesterol-lowering arm of the study in October 2002, nearly two years earlier than planned.

Pfizer trumpeted this fact from the rooftops at the time, implying that atorvastatin was just so damned wonderful that the benefits had emerged in double-quick time. This made it unethical not to give the drug. All very fine and noble and public spirited, no doubt.

What was not shouted from the rooftops was the total mortality data. Indeed, in analyses of the trial it wasn't mentioned at all. Here is one example. It's a bit long, and gigantically dull, but I just want to make the point that benefit after benefit is being highlighted here, yet there is nothing about total mortality:

Follow-up was planned for an average of 5 years. The ASCOT-LLA was stopped after 3.3 years owing to the superiority of atorvastatin 10 mg over placebo in reducing the primary end point of nonfatal myocardial infarction (MI) and fatal CHD... Cholesterol lowering with atorvastatin was associated with a highly significant reduction in the primary end point of nonfatal MI and fatal CHD (36%, P = 0.0005). The observed benefit was consistent across the secondary end points and the 18 prespecified subgroups. The ASCOT-LLA findings have influenced lipid-lowering guidelines and support the concept that treatment strategies to reduce cardiovascular disease should be based on the assessment of all cardiovascular risk factors, rather than on numerical thresholds of individual risk factors, to determine treatment strategies.'

Am J Med, December 2005; 118 Suppl 12A

In the case of ASCOT-LLA, however, the total mortality data were published. So I took the graph of overall mortality, scanned it, and I have reproduced it for you in (Fig. 27). The dotted line represents deaths in the placebo group, the solid line represents deaths in the atorvastatin group.

Fig. 27 Total mortality: atorvastatin vs placebo

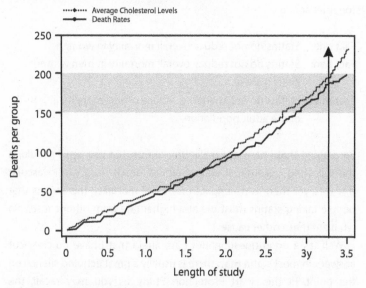

I also did something else to this graph. I added in my own line at 3.3 years. I did this because the trial actually ended at 3.3 years. Yet, as you may notice, the data lines dribble on for another three months. The study was stopped, yet the data analysis went on?

Why did this happen? Well, perhaps it is relevant to point out that that from 3.3 years to 3.5 years the total mortality lines divide sharply in favour of atorvastatin (the only time period when this happened). At 3.3 years, there was hardly any discernible difference between drug and placebo, yet by 3.5 years there were 185 deaths in the atorvastatin group and 212 in the placebo group.

This difference still did not manage to limp its way to statistical significance, but it was considerably better than the difference three months earlier, which was approximately zero. By the way, I haven't got the exact figures for 3.3 years. I have asked for them, but silence was the stern reply. I have also asked the authors how a trial can end after 3.3 years, yet data collection continues for another 3 months – 'unblinded' and uncontrolled. Silence.

However, at this stage I think it's worth pulling two or three facts together again:

Fact one: Statins do not reduce overall mortality in women.
Fact two: Statins do not reduce overall mortality in men without heart disease.
Fact three: Statins do not, therefore, reduce overall morality in > 95% of the adult population.

Something that I have not really brought up, but perhaps I should, is the following question. If statins reduce death from cardiovascular diseases, yet there is no impact on overall mortality, this means that people taking statins must die at a higher rate from other causes. So what are these other causes?

Well, it's a good question. But I am afraid that I have no clear-cut answers. In most statin trials there is usually a great echoing silence on the point. In the Heart Protection Study, as you may recall, the researchers didn't even bother to publish the overall mortality data in women, let alone list exactly what people died of. This type of thing makes it rather difficult to get a handle on what people who are taking statins die of instead of heart disease. The data just ain't there.

This area is made even more opaque by the reaction of the mainstream researchers to overall mortality data. A recent statin study called 'Treat to New Targets (TNT)', failed – once again – to show any benefit on total mortality. According to head researcher of the TNT study, Dr John LaRosa, *'We need to make the assumption that mortality has been proven, that LDL lowering does in fact lower total mortality rates.'* We need to the make the assumption? Why does a researcher need to make assumptions – especially when all the evidence seems to me to point the other way?

Dr Roger Blumenthal, from Johns Hopkins University Medical Center, in Baltimore, Maryland, said that the TNT mortality finding was *'unfortunate'* and *'a bit surprising'*, but that the increase in non-cardiovascular mortality was 'likely due to chance'. Blumenthal went on to claim that, '*The totality of evidence does not suggest that lowering LDL cholesterol to very low levels is associated with non-cardiovascular mortality.*' If there were fewer cardiovascular deaths in the TNT trial, yet no difference in overall mortality, I would have thought that there is only one conclusion that can be drawn: there were more non-cardiovascular deaths.

At this point, hopefully, you are beginning to realise that statins may not be quite as super-wonderful as you may have thought. You may also be wondering how it is that, despite their almost complete lack of any real benefit – i.e. actually saving lives – statins have been hyped to the very skies. There is a very simple reason for this. It's called money.

Rosuvastatin (Crestor) was launched a couple of years ago, or so. In the first year of its launch, $1 billion was spent on sales and marketing. To quote Dr Evil from *Austin Powers*: 'One… beellion… dollars.' And this, remember, was only the budget for one of the six statins on the market. One…. beellion…. dollars, it must be said, buys a hell of a lot of publicity.

At the same time, you could pay journalists to attend international meetings, and provide them with PR company-generated press packs highlighting the wonders of your drug. Positive findings can then be hyped relentlessly, and the health editors of newspapers wined and dined. Ghost authors can then be found to write up the findings of trials, ensuring that the correct marketing spin is applied to the data. Opinion leaders lend their imprimatur to the papers at the end of this process – along with an eye-watering invoice, naturally.

Nowadays, the entire world of clinical trials is controlled to a quite extraordinary degree. To quote Dr Marcia Angell, who used to edit the *New England Journal of Medicine* (which is one of the top five most influential medical journals in the world – possibly even number one):

> *It used to be that drug companies simply gave grants to academic medical centres for the use of their clinical researchers to do a study and that was it. It was at arm's length. The researcher did a study and he or she published the results,*

whatever those results would be. Now, it's very, very different. The drug companies increasingly design the studies. They keep the data. They don't even let the researchers see the data. They analyse the data, they decide whether they're going to even publish the data at the end of it. They sign contracts with researchers and with academic medical centres saying that they don't get to publish their work unless they get permission from the drug company. So, you can see that the distortion starts even before publication. It starts in determining what's going to be published and what isn't going to be published. This is no longer arm's length. It's treating the researchers and the academic medical centres as though they were hired guns or technicians or something. They just do the work. And the drug company will decide what the data show, what the conclusions are and whether it will even be published.

In short, the medical profession is increasingly working closely with pharmaceutical companies.

If you have no role in major pharmaceutical-sponsored clinical trials then you do not speak at major meetings, you do not publish 'prestige' papers in high-impact journals, you do not bring in money to your university department. You have little to offer at major international conferences. You live in Backwatersville, man.

A Dr John Kastelein from Amsterdam was utterly outraged that anyone should have objected to the last set of NCEP guidelines because of potential conflicts. He felt that the whole conflict-of-interest issue was being over-hyped. In his words:

I don't believe a word about the conflict of interest because there is no single opinion leader in the world who has not done any work for a pharmaceutical company in terms of research or trials.

He is supported in his stance by Harvard Medical School Associate Professor Daniel Simon. In his view it's a mistake to tune out the views of those with potential conflicts of interest because the pharmaceutical industry is driving medical advances. Most unconflicted researchers 'are not truly expert'. He says.

In an attempt to get some handle on potential conflicts of interest, several of the most prestigious medical journals banded together to demand that those involved in clinical trials, or writing editorials, reveal their connections to the pharmaceutical industry. This is a process known as 'disclosure'.

To my mind, there are some major problems with disclosure. The first is that if you do not 'disclose', absolutely nothing happens – at all. This may not be a victimless crime, but it most certainly is a 'punishmentless' crime. If you are rumbled, you can just do a Bill Clinton: 'But what is disclosure, exactly. Oh, I misunderstood... sorry. You mean being paid vast sums of money by a pharmaceutical company should be disclosed? Gosh. Who would have thought? Golly, I'll try to remember in the future... promise.'

Entering the debate, the NCEP have said:

> The members of experts panels charged with developing guidelines are selected for their scientific and medical expertise, their stature and track record in the field, and their integrity. Individuals who are most expert in a subject area are the ones most suitable to serve on a guideline panel for assessing the science and developing clinical recommendations. They are also often the very people whose advice is sought by industry. Most guideline panels therefore include experts who interact with industry ...

I especially liked the bit about integrity, though. How did they measure this? Did they buy a new Acme integrityometer, only £29.99 from Argos? Or did they get all the panel members to eat beans and go up and down in a lift, checking that whoever broke wind owned up each time? Panel members selected for their 'stature and track record in the field, and their integrity', is otherwise known as Eminence Based Medicine (EBM).

Eric Topol, just to give one more example, maintains that he has severed his ties with the industry in 2004. Here's a little something on the matter from his website www.theheart.org:

> Topol is unique in that he extricated all ties with industry in 2004. 'I do not believe that my historical relationship with companies with financial interests in this area is influencing patient care today. I have never ordered a commercial test for aspirin or Plavix resistance for any patient and never advocated the use of such tests for clinical care,' he writes, adding that it was not mentioned that he published the only article in a peer-reviewed journal warning physicians of the unanticipated potential conflicts of interest in relationships with the investment industry. 'I have taken a very hard stance on the troubles of the academia-industry megacomplex, have repeatedly challenged industry when there was any question of potential public-health harm, and have tried to set an example of dissociation from industry while still performing important research to advance heart-disease prevention and therapy. It is ironic that an article that purports to unveil bias among physicians besmirches me.'

Again, I will have to leave it up to you to sit on the internet for an afternoon and read the facts that my publisher is reluctant to publish.

If you do so virtually you will find links between all prominent cardiologists and the pharmaceutical industry.

I know that all opinion leaders would be shocked and outraged if you were to suggest to them that they were in any way influenced by the money that they earn from the industry. They consider themselves paragons of virtue. On this issue, however, I defer to the great Robbie Burns:

> O wad some Power the giftie gie us,
> To see oursels as ithers see us!
> It wad frae mony a blunder free us.

THE DAMAGE THAT STATINS CAN DO

Moving on from their complete lack of any benefits – for the vast majority of the population – the next thing to mention is the serious damage that statins are already doing to the NHS budget. Currently, they are the most expensive single item of drug expenditure. While the figures keep on changing, in the very near future, if it has not already happened, statins will cost the NHS over £1 billion per year.

But this is only the costs of the drugs themselves. There are many additional costs:

- Yearly cholesterol tests
- Six-month review by a GP, or nurse
- Payment to GPs for getting blood cholesterol levels down through the Quality Outcome Framework system

Just to tease out one figure in more detail. If we consider that ten million people, at the very least, are supposed to be on statins and they are given a six-month check-up, this amounts to twenty million consultations per year. An average consultation, adding in blood tests, doctor's time, payment for QoF payment etc., is at least £50, absolute minimum. So this is an extra £1 billion, on top of the £1 billion spent on the statins.

Two billion pounds a year is a not inconsiderable sum of money. What else could you do with the money? Well, you could employ around 70,000 extra nurses a year to start with, which isn't bad going. Or build two brand, spanking new university-sized hospitals, fully equipped, each year. Take your pick.

But you know. A billion here, two billion there – it's only money, after all. What I am more interested in looking at here is the potential physical harm that statins can do – apart from possibly causing horribly deformed babies, of course.

At this point, I should state that I do not think that statins are hugely dangerous. In most of the trials statins, have done nothing at all to improve overall mortality, but they don't seem to have increased the death rate. So putting someone on a statin is unlikely to actually kill them. Having said this, of course, statins may kill. Cerivastatin, the drug withdrawn by Bayer, was implicated in the deaths of at least 100 people before it got withdrawn. Data from the FDA show that simvastatin was established as a direct cause of death in 416 people between 1997 and 2004. All statins have been linked directly to people dying. How many exactly? Who knows? How could you know?

Vioxx, the arthritis drug, was estimated to have been linked to more than 100,000 deaths in the USA in two years. And no one noticed! The fatal effects of Vioxx were only picked up coincidentally as part of a major trial to see if this drug could protect against bowel cancer. The impact on mortality was noted, and highlighted, by a rather heroic employee of the Food and Drugs Administration (FDA), Dr David Graham. For his efforts in protecting the safety of the public he was smeared in the press and ruthlessly attacked. Luckily, a certain Senator Charles Grassley got involved in the case. He wrote a letter to Lester Crawford, the acting commissioner at the FDA at the time. I reprint some sections of it here, because it is an absolute cracker. A symphony in restrained rage:

> As Chairman of the Committee on Finance, I have made it clear to you that I expect that Dr David Graham's right as a federal employee will be fully respected by the Food and Drug Administration. Last Wednesday, November 24, 2004, I requested that the Office of Inspector General (OIG), Department of Health and Human Services conduct a complete and thorough investigation into the facts, events, persons, policies, regulations and laws relating to allegations that a number of management level employees at the FDA may have acted 'to discredit an outspoken agency safety office who was challenging the FDA's drug safety policies.' I referred to the attached article from the Washington Post entitled, 'Attempt to Discredit Whistle-Blower Alleged.'...

I'd like to reiterate what I have repeatedly stated in writing and have verbally communicated to your agency, namely that this Committee takes its responsibility to protect witnesses and particularly government witnesses very seriously, and that holds particularly true for Dr Graham.'...

I understand that retaliatory action against dissident employees can come under many guises. Therefore, I also request that you address allegations that administrative action may be taken against Dr Graham, including that he may be terminated or transferred against his wishes to a job other than conducting scientific research. Please advise me whether there is any truth to these allegations and, if so, explain what actions are being taken to transfer Dr Graham from his present position and duties at FDA...
On at least 6 separate occasions – 3 by letter and 3 in meetings with FDA staff – I have requested that FDA employees be advised that they may come to Congress and speak freely without fear of reprisal. Do you believe that FDA employees are free to speak to members of Congress without advising FDA's Office of Legislation? If so, when are you going to act on this request?

Ouch!

This sorry saga highlights that fact that a drug could potentially kill hundreds of thousands of people without anyone actually noticing. You may think that this must be impossible. There have to be agencies out there monitoring this sort of thing on a day-to-day basis, combing through the statistics with a fine-tooth comb? Not so – and anyway, how could they? Drug safety is supposed to be fully established in the clinical trial process. Once a drug is out there in the community it could wipe out thousands, unnoticed – witness Vioxx.

In addition to the difficulty of expecting an individual doctor to spot patterns of increased mortality, the majority of people taking statins are usually taking other drugs at the same time. So how can anyone know which drug did what? And what's more, very few doctors report adverse events at all.

In short, although it seems unlikely that statins are killing thousands of people, it's as well to remain vigilant. After all, it could take a long time for serious effects to emerge – much longer than any of the statin trials have lasted. Five years may seem sufficient to pick up on serious effects, but if you ran a five-year clinical study on the effects of smoking, you would see no impact on lung cancer – at all. Statins, potentially, are going to be taken for 30, 40, 50 years. Are they safe over this time period? Only time will tell.

Moving on to more immediate effects. The primary way that statins kill people is through a side effect known as rhabdomyolysis, which is breakdown of skeletal muscle. Basically, your muscles dissolve away, the waste products from this process destroy the kidneys and you can then die from kidney failure. This, I hasten to add, is not common. According to one report, in the USA over two and a half years there were only 871 reports of rhabdomyolysis with statins, 38 of which were fatal. How many more cases went unreported is unknown, although several studies have calculated that adverse event reporting underestimates the true number of events by about 95 per cent. Even so, this is not an epidemic by any means.

The major problem with statins though, is not that they kill a few hundred people here and there, it is that they create a huge burden of insidious side effects, most of which go unnoticed, or are dismissed. You feel tired? Well, you are getting older, after all. Muscle pains? Hell, we all get them. Even when you suffer a complete belter of a side effect, most doctors refuse to believe this could possibly have anything to do with the statin you are taking.

Let me introduce you to a doctor in the USA called Duane Graveline. He is a family doctor, but he also trained as an astronaut with NASA, and works closely with airline pilots to assess their fitness to fly. Some years ago, he was found to have a raised cholesterol level and was put on a statin. He had no problem with this, as he fully believed in the cholesterol hypothesis and the benefits of statins.

However, he then suffered a highly disturbing episode of memory loss, so he stopped taking the statin. He had no further problems for the next year, so his doctor persuaded him start a statin again, and he did so. Shortly after this, he suffered a much worse episode of memory loss, during which he regressed into his teenage years, unable to recall training as a doctor at all. After regaining his memory he was very shaken by the whole episode and binned the statins for good.

The doctors treating him made the diagnosis of transient global amnesia, cause unknown. They totally refused to accept the possibility that the statin could be the cause, and neither would anyone else. Feeling like a lonely voice in the wilderness, Dr Graveline then published a letter on a website called People's Pharmacy asking if anyone else taking statins had suffered the same thing. He was immediately inundated by hundreds of cases from distraught patients and relatives. They described a full array of cognitive side effects from amnesia and severe memory loss to confusion and disorientation – all associated with statins, mostly with atorvastatin (Lipitor). The response of the mainstream medical community, however, could be paraphrased thus: 'You don't know what you're talking about. Statins are safe and have very few side effects.'

Here is one letter that was written to Dr Graveline and is reproduced in his book *Lipitor, Thief of Memory*:

> *About six weeks ago, my doctor doubled my Lipitor from 20 milligrams to 40 milligrams. For about the past four weeks I have experienced progressive memory loss. I couldn't remember my brother's phone number. I couldn't find my baby's plate of food after preparing it. I couldn't remember recent trips. I couldn't remember to attend a meeting. I couldn't remember a restaurant I ate in and numerous other similar episodes. This is totally out of character for me. I have called my doctor and am awaiting his return call. For your information I am 39 years old and have been on Lipitor about four years.*

Will this be memory loss be ignored by the doctor? Probably. Will this be filed as an adverse event? Almost certainly not. This effect will be considered trivial. However, I think that the 'mental' problems associated with statins are far from trivial. As early as the 1960s it was recognised that the people taking cholesterol-lowering drugs tended to die more frequently from violent deaths: accidents, suicide, shootings and the like. This was universally dismissed as a coincidental finding (no matter how many times it cropped up), mainly because no one was able to see how a low cholesterol level could possibly be linked to violent deaths.

I read one post-hoc analysis of a cholesterol-lowering trial in which the authors were so determined to prove that the low cholesterol levels could have nothing to do with dying in a car crash that they pushed the analytical boundaries into another dimension. Their argument was that several of those who died while on statins were actually pedestrians, not drivers. So the statin couldn't be to blame for the crash. Ha! Just try picking the logic out of that statement.

Anyway, thirty years ago, even twenty years ago, even five years ago, no one knew that cholesterol had anything to do with brain function. This despite that fact that the brain contains over 25 per cent of the total amount of cholesterol in the body, and over 2 per cent of the total weight of the brain is cholesterol (presumably it was thought to be hanging about in the brain by accident?). However, it has more recently been discovered that if you want the brain to function, this requires cholesterol.

A group of researchers, led by Dr Frank Pfrieger, was looking into the function of glial cells in the brain. It was known that these 'support' cells had a critical role in the function of synapses (the connections between neurons). Glial cells, it was also known, released a substance that allowed synapses to form, and function. Without this substance your brain would be almost entirely useless. And what was this fantastic, miracle substance?

> *Isolated neurons in the laboratory survived and grew, but showed only a few of the electrical signals generated by synapses. But*

> *when exposed to substances secreted by glial cells they produced*
> *strong signs of synaptic activity. The identity of the glial ingredient*
> *which triggered synapse formation has remained a mystery until*
> *now. But research published in the journal* Science *suggests that*
> *cholesterol is the magic ingredient.*

Yes, the magic ingredient was good old 'deadly' cholesterol. Without cholesterol, the chemical scourge of mankind, your brain cannot form synapses, and you can't think properly, or remember anything. Or remember anything.

Maybe it was a tad premature to write off cognitive side effects as a mere coincidence? Especially when it is clear how taking a statin might, just might, cause memory loss, even global amnesia. In fact, it is hard to see how it would not. It might also be possible to see how you would be more likely to die in a car crash – either as a driver or pedestrian – if your brain isn't functioning properly. 'Now, do I look left, or right?'

But what about the link between cholesterol lowering, violence, and suicide? Well, in addition to cholesterol's critical function in synapse formation, it has now been found that a low cholesterol level leads to reduced serotonin levels in the brain. A low serotonin level is one of the key brain abnormalities involved in depression. This is why the most commonly used anti-depressants are designed to boost serotonin levels. They are known as Selective Serotonin Re-Uptake Inhibitors (SSRIs). Prozac is the most famous of this group of drugs.

Low serotonin has also been linked to violence and aggression. And this is far from a theoretical finding. A group of researchers led by Jian Zhang looked at the association between a low cholesterol level and a history of school suspension. They concluded that:

> *Among non-African-American children, low total cholesterol is*
> *associated with school suspension or expulsion and that low total*
> *cholesterol may be a risk factor for aggression or a risk marker for*
> *other biologic variables that predispose to aggression.*

... the results of the current study are consistent with the majority of previous studies examining the associations between low serum cholesterol and various forms of aggression in adults. With few exceptions significant associations have been observed from cross-sectional studies, cohort samples, general population studies, psychiatric patients and criminals, and controlled dietary studies conducted in nonhuman primates. In particular, low total cholesterol has been associated with the onset of conduct disorder during childhood among male criminals.

Added to this, the Royal College of Psychiatry published a paper looking at the role of cholesterol in depression and self harm. It was entitled 'Low cholesterol may indicate risk of suicide'. Here I take a few sections from the press release:

Lower cholesterol levels were related to higher levels of self-reported impulsivity. The finding of a lower average cholesterol in the DSH (Depression and Self Harm) group confirms other published studies.

The authors hypothesise that the increased death rates in populations with low cholesterol may be the result of increased suicide and accident rates associated with increased tendencies to impulsivity.

It may be that low cholesterol in some way influences the function of the central nervous system, or acts as a marker for factors governing a predisposition to death by trauma and suicide.

It is thought that cholesterol may influence serotonin, a neurotransmitter in the brain, low levels of which are associated not only with depression and suicide, but also with aggression and impulsivity. The latter are often involved before accidents, acts of violence to self and others and attempted or completed suicide.

And so, gentle reader, our scientific knowledge has now advanced to the point where it can no longer be written off as a 'coincidence' that people on cholesterol-lowering drugs are more likely to die violent deaths of one sort or another. A clear causal chain now exists, with every link in place.

As a little postscript to this section I would like to quote Frank Pfrieger again: '*A defective cholesterol metabolism in the brain may impair its development and function.*' So it may also not be a coincidence that you can get serious neurological abnormalities in babies whose mothers were taking statins while pregnant.

How widespread are all of these problems? Who knows? If they exist they will be, almost without exception, underreported. A bit of memory loss here, a lapse into depression there – well, everyone is depressed nowadays, aren't they? Feelings of anger and aggression, a bit of road rage, some muscle pains. Which patient is going to report such symptoms to their GP? And even if they do, how seriously is the GP going to take it? Remember that Dr Graveline suffered a full-blown episode of global amnesia and he was still hounded to re-start his statins.

What are the other problems with statins? For the sake of brevity, I shall run through them at relatively high speed.

Polyneuropathy
Polyneuropathy, also known as peripheral neuropathy, is characterised by the following:

- Facial weakness
- Difficulty in walking
- Difficulty using the arms, hands, or feet
- Sensation changes (usually of the arms and hands or legs and feet), such as pain, burning, tingling, numbness or decreased sensation
- Difficulty swallowing
- Speech impairment
- Loss of muscle function or feeling in the muscles

- Pain in the joints
- Hoarseness or changing of voice
- Fatigue

Researchers who studied half a million people in Denmark found that those who took statins were significantly more likely to develop polyneuropathy. Just how significantly was highlighted by a study published by the American Academy of Neurology. The researchers found that patients treated with statins for two or more years had a 26.4-fold increase in the risk of definite idiopathic (caused by a drug) polyneuropathy. That is a 2,640 per cent increase in risk.

In general, polyneuropathy is irreversible.

Muscle damage
Although rhabdomyolysis itself is rare, muscle pains and muscle weakness are relatively common with statin use. It is very difficult to get a handle on how common this is. The mainstream view is that about one per cent of people taking statins will suffer muscle pain, or weakness.

However, I have seen much higher figures. Dr James K Liao, director of vascular medicine research at Brigham & Women's Hospital in Boston and a big supporter of statins, believes muscle pains are much more common, occurring in 15 per cent to 20 per cent of his patients.

In this world, as with much else, seek and ye shall find. A research group in Austria decided to analyse 111 people with FH who had been put on statins, and complained of no side effects whatsoever. But the researchers wanted to know if there were signs of muscle injury anyway. They used a test that is not widely available, but is the gold standard for detecting 'oxidative' damage. (They measured 8-epi-prostaglandin PGF2alpha, if you really want to know.) To their surprise, they found that 11 of the subjects had significant biochemical signs of oxidative damage to their muscles.

> *These findings indicate that in the absence of other clinically observable adverse effects, in some of the patients, for an as yet*

> unknown reason, statin therapy may be associated with increased
> oxidation injury.

Is this clinically important? Who knows? Maybe not for everyone. But this same group of Austrian researchers discovered that statin-related muscle problems are much more likely to occur in those who do a lot of exercise. They looked at a group of professional athletes with FH and found that only 20 per cent of them could tolerate using statins without suffering serious muscle pain and weakness.

Apart from athletes, I am certain that the burden of muscle problems is generally underestimated because such problems tend to creep up slowly. My father in-law takes statins – don't worry, he wouldn't dream of listening to me. (Although maybe he will after reading this damned book...) After his statin dose was increased last year he was unable to walk more than a hundred yards without having to sit down and rest. He was persuaded to reduce the dose, and he can now walk for over a mile, easily. Of course neither he nor his doctor believe that his muscle weakness and pain was in any way related to the increased statin dose. After all, he is approaching eighty, he has had a heart attack, he was already slowing down. So what do you expect? We are all remarkably good at dismissing the symptoms of others.

Personally, I believe that a very high percentage of people on statins will suffer some symptoms of muscle ache; most of them they won't report the symptoms, and the doctor won't ask. Doctors are not generally very keen on discovering problems with the drugs that they prescribe.

Liver damage

This is reasonably common, although in the main not serious. Mostly it takes the form of raised liver-enzyme levels in the bloodstream. These tend to go away when you stop taking the statin. There have been cases of liver failure while on statins, but these are relatively rare.

Cancer

This is probably the biggest long-term worry as far as I am concerned. To quote a study from the *Journal of the American Medical Association* published in 1996:

> *All members of the two most popular classes of lipid-lowering drugs (the fibrates and the statins) cause cancer in rodents, in some cases at levels of animal exposure close to those prescribed to humans...*
>
> *Extrapolation of this evidence of carcinogenesis from rodents to humans is an uncertain process. Longer-term clinical trials and careful postmarketing surveillance during the next several decades are needed to determine whether cholesterol-lowering drugs cause cancer in humans. In the meantime, the results of experiments in animals and humans suggest that lipid-lowering drug treatment, especially with the fibrates and statins, should be avoided except in patients at high short-term risk of coronary heart disease.*

The pharmaceutical companies have attempted to stomp on this fear by setting up studies that appear to show that statins, rather than causing cancer, actually prevent it. Attack, as they say, is the best form of defence. You may have seen some of the headlines, such as:

> *New research shows that the popular cholesterol-lowering drugs called statins may slash a person's chance of developing breast, prostate, and lung tumors in half.*

I plucked the above headline from a major medical website called WebMD. So what's actually wrong with this 'new research'? Let's put it this way:

- People with low cholesterol levels are at a much greater risk of dying of cancer.
- People with low cholesterol levels don't get put on statins (yet).

However,

- People with high cholesterol levels are less likely to die of cancer.
- People with high cholesterol levels do get put on statins.

Therefore, if you find a group of people taking statins, and match them against a group of people not taking statins, hey presto! It is very likely you will see less cancer in those taking statins, because they were protected against cancer in the first place.

Luckily, it doesn't actually take long to stomp such headlines into the ground. In the major statin trials, the people taking the statins and those taking the placebo are allocated at random, so on average both groups should have identical cholesterol levels. And guess what? When a meta-analysis of the statin trials was done, and published in JAMA, looking for any effect on cancer:

> *In our current meta-analysis, statins did not reduce the incidence of cancer or cancer death, No reductions were noted for cancers of the breast, colon, gastrointestinal tract, prostate, respiratory tract, or skin (melanoma) when statins were used... the patients in our meta-analysis were primarily treated with simvastatin and pravastatin. As such, we evaluated pravastatin alone and simvastatin alone on cancer incidence and death and found no impact.*

In short, the headlines about statins preventing cancer are complete and utter guff, as usual. They reflect marketing spin, pure and simple. But they do their job, the message gets out there: statins don't cause cancer, they actually protect against cancer. Goodness me, is there nothing these drugs can't do?

So, while there is no evidence that statins protect against cancer, is there any evidence that they may increase the risk of cancer? There is some, but it is fragmented. A massive (and never-remarked-upon) statin trial in Japan, the J-LIT study, found a small proportion of patients who were 'hyper-responders' to simvastatin, i.e. their LDL levels fell dramatically when given the drug. In this group there was a significant increase in deaths from cancer.

In addition to this, in the PROSPER study – one of the few statin trials specifically carried out on older people (for whom cancer risk is increased) – there were 24 more cases of cancer in the statin arm than the placebo arm. This, by the way, more than cancelled out all cardiovascular benefits. In the CARE study there were 12 cases of breast cancer in the statin arm against one in the placebo arm.

None of this is definitive proof that statins cause cancer, by any manner of means. But to my mind, it is something that needs to be carefully monitored. After all, we already have a few disturbing facts at our disposal:

- Statins cause cancer in animals.
- There is some evidence that cancer deaths are increased in the statin trials, especially in those who are 'hyper-responders' to statins.
- A low cholesterol level is associated with a high risk of death from cancer.
- It can take many, many years for cancer-causing agents to reveal themselves.

I think that this is more than enough evidence to warrant a high degree of suspicion. So is anyone studying this in any meaningful way? You must be joking. It would be like asking British American Tobacco to fund a study into nicotine addiction.

Heart failure

There are actually a myriad of other statin-related side effects. But you would expect to see this in any drug that was being taken by millions of people. A couple that seem to turn up more regularly than others are acute pancreatitis and severe dizziness. However, there is one potentially very worrying side effect that I would like to draw your attention to, heart failure.

In the late 1980s, when Merck were first readying themselves to launch their two statins – lovastatin (Mevacor) followed by simvastatin (Zocor) – they applied for a patent in which their statins would be combined with a substance known as coenzyme Q10. A substance that, for the sake of brevity, I will call Q10 from now on.

Q10 is found in all cells, everywhere in the body, which is why it is sometimes called ubiquinone (because is it ubiquitous). It is found in particularly high concentrations in high-energy cells such as muscles, and especially cardiac muscle cells, where it plays a key role in the production of ATP. ATP, as you may remember from biology, is to a cell, what fuel is to a car. Conversion of ATP to ADP releases the energy that cells need to work. When ATP runs out, the cell dies. Which means that a reduction in ATP production could be a rather serious matter. Especially in heart muscle, the muscle that can never rest. Indeed, both animal and human studies have shown that reduced Q10 levels can lead to left- and right-sided ventricular dysfunction (heart failure to you and me).

So where is all this going, you may ask. Well, at this point I shall draw another strand into the discussion. You see, Q10 and cholesterol share a biosynthetic pathway. They both originate from Acetyl CoA, and if you block HMG CoA reductase you not only reduce cholesterol synthesis, you also reduce Q10 synthesis. The two pathways do not split until after this point.

If low Q10 levels can lead to heart failure, and statins block the production of Q10, then statins could cause heart failure. Thus, adding Q10 to a statin makes perfect sense, does it not? In the end, though, Merck never acted on their patents (patent 4929437, issued 29 May 1990 and US Patent 4933165, issued 12 June 1990, both entitled 'Coenzyme Q10 with HMG-CoA Reductase Inhibitors'). Why not? Well, this is the sort of 'commercially sensitive' information that Merck have not published. I note, however, that:

• Combination pills are more expensive to make, and it takes longer to get approval from the authorities to launch them.

- Adding Q10 to a statin might be an admission that statins are not totally innocent, cuddly and safe – could they be if they required a built-in 'antidote'?
- Other statins coming to the market were not going to add Q10 to their statin.
- The risk of causing heart failure in humans by lowering Q10 levels had not been definitively proven.

Having said this, Merck may have been worried enough by something they had seen to fill in two separate patents for a combination pill, a most unusual move. Their research remains unpublished, so I can only speculate on what it showed.

As a little aside, it may be pertinent to this discussion to point out that Merck also make (or should that be made) Vioxx. While they claimed that the increased risk of heart attacks came as a complete surprise to them when this finding first 'appeared' in late 2004, during the course of three lawsuits against Merck, it was alleged they deliberately witheld data on the cardiavascular dangers of the drug. You can read about this on the Forbes website:
http://www.forbes.com/markets/2005/12/08/merck-vioxx-study 1208markets14.html

Moving on. In addition to the possibility that statins could cause heart failure by blocking Q10 synthesis, a study published in the 3 December 2003 edition of the *Journal of the American College of Cardiology* reported a strong relationship between lower cholesterol levels and increased mortality in patients with heart failure. The study was conducted in the Royal Brompton Chronic Heart Failure Clinic in London. The researchers measured cholesterol levels in over 400 patients with varying degrees of heart failure and followed their outcomes. They found that people with cholesterol levels below 5.0mmol/l have a two- to three-fold increased risk of dying compared to those whose cholesterol levels were higher. In fact, it has been noted in many studies that heart-failure patients seem to have 'reverse epidemiology'. By this, I mean that having a high cholesterol level and being obese and having a high blood pressure are associated with prolonged survival.

Bringing all of the strands together, it seems that there are two interrelated mechanisms by which statins could cause heart failure. Firstly, by blocking Q10, thus lowering the heart-muscle energy production; secondly, by lowering cholesterol levels. The 'Coenzyme Q10 Association' (yes, there is one) were worried enough about this to have written to the FDA expressing their concern. I believe that they are awaiting a reply – I would advise them not to hold their breath.

There are also cardiologists out there who believe that the current sharp rise in heart failure across the western world is a direct result of the use of statins. Theoretically, at least, they have a strong point. However, I don't believe that the data yet exists to prove the case one way or the other. Once again, though, there is enough evidence out there to warrant close attention and monitoring.

A final thought:

- Several studies have shown that a low cholesterol level is a major risk factor for people with heart failure.
- Statins significantly reduce the risk of death once you have heart failure.

So, in this case, statins must be working through *non* cholesterol-lowering effects.

And finally – the damage that statins can do
Leaving aside physical side effects and the eye-watering cost, the ever-increasing use of statins will have, I believe, a major negative impact on society as a whole.

To give just one example of the potential scale of the impact, a couple of years ago a group of researchers in Norway looked at the latest guidelines on CHD prevention published by the European Society of Cardiology. They wanted to see what the full implementation of these guidelines would mean for the Norwegian population – a population which, as the authors point out – has an average life expectancy of 79 – making it one of the longest lived in the history of mankind.

The European guidelines defined a blood pressure of 140/90, and a cholesterol level of 5.0mmo/l, as thresholds for intervention. (Intervention means, in 99 per cent of cases, drug treatment.) Using these two levels, the Norwegian researchers then drew a graph showing what percentage of the population would be in the 'at risk' category for high cholesterol and/or a raised blood pressure (see below):

Fig. 28 Drug treatment levels per age group

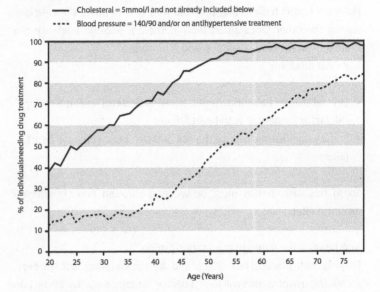

As you can see, by the age of 25, 50 per cent of the population is 'at risk' from their high cholesterol levels. By the age of 50 this has gone up to 90 per cent. And if you in add raised blood pressure, there is hardly anyone left who does not require 'intervention'.

What's implied here is that the majority of Norwegians are so unhealthy that they need drug treatment. And, although no one has done it yet, if you applied these latest European guidelines to the UK, you would find an even higher percentage requiring life-long drug treatment.

In my view, this is about as far from the concept of health as it is possible to get. We are in grave danger of converting the vast majority of adults in the country from 'healthy', to 'diseased', and worried to boot. And the only solution for your 'disease'? Take a statin for the rest of your life, and never stop.

Can it really be true that 90 per cent of the population need life-long medication? This is bonkers. It is *Brave New World*, it is a combination of all dystopian nightmares of the future come to life. Health, it would seem, is no longer an absence of disease, but an absence of taking the correct medication.

First, do no harm? I don't think so.

Statins don't work by lowering LDL levels

At this point, grudgingly, I will admit that statins do reduce the risk of dying of heart disease in certain populations. Statins definitely reduce overall mortality in men with existing heart disease. So, if you are a man with known heart disease, it may be a good idea to take a statin. (There, I said it – and it did hurt, thanks for asking.) However, before looking at how they actually do this, I think you ought to know in a bit more detail what the figures are.

Here I include a chart copied from Uffe Ravnskov, who wrote the book *The Cholesterol Myths*, and with whom I communicate regularly. He looked at overall mortality rates from the six biggest statin trials at the time and brought together four different figures related to overall mortality.

- The relative risk reduction
- The absolute risk reduction
- The chances of being alive at the end of the trial on placebo
- The chances of being alive at the end of the trial on a statin

Risk reduction (total mortality) in six clinical statin trials

	Relative risk	Absolute risk	Chance of surviving on placebo	Chance of surviving on statin
4S	-29%	-3.3%	88.5%	91.8%
WOSCOPS	-21%	-0.9%	95.9%	96.8%
CARE	-8%	-0.78%	90.57%	91.35%
AFCAPS/TexCAPS	+3.9%	+0.09%	97.7%	97.6%
LIPID	-21%	-3.1%	85.9%	89.0%
EXCEL	+150%	+0.3%	99.8%	99.5%

These figures represent a mixture of primary and secondary prevention. The reason for using them is to give you an idea of the general scale of risk reductions found in the statin trials. Let's concentrate on three of them in a little more detail: 4S, WOSCOPS and EXCEL.

The 4S trial remains the most positive of all the statin trials. In this study, there was a 3.3 per cent absolute risk reduction in total mortality over five years, which equates to a 0.66 per cent reduction in overall mortality each year. This was purely a secondary prevention trial.

WOCSOPS was a mixed primary/secondary prevention study. However, average cholesterol levels in this trial were 7.0mmol/l, which puts everyone in the study into a 'high risk' category. In WOSCOPS there was a 0.9 per cent reduction in overall mortality over five years – which represents a 0.18 per cent reduction in overall mortality per year.

Just to present the other side of the story, in the EXCEL trial, which was entirely a primary prevention study, there was a 0.3 per cent increase in overall mortality over five years. Once again, perhaps these figures are not quite as spectacular as you would imagine, given the hype that surrounds statins.

Before moving on from the statistics, I would like to tackle the use of the term 'saving lives'. You may remember the press release that accompanied the HPS study:

If now, as a result, an extra 10 million high-risk people were to go onto statin treatment, this would save about 50,000 lives a year – that's a thousand each week.

Leaving aside the point that this 50,000 figure actually equates to one life 'saved' for every 200 people taking the statin – 10 million is an awful lot of people to use as your denominator – the concept of saving lives, suggesting, as it does, that each of the 50,000 whose lives have been saved will go on to live out a full and healthy life, is not best chosen.

In reality, taking a statin can only delay death, not prevent it. By how much? Well, if one in two hundred more people are alive after one year of taking statins, this means that if you wait another two-hundredths of a year (plus another little bit) the statin group will have caught up on the 'placebo' group in total number of deaths. This represents an increased life expectancy of slightly under two days.

So, rather than stating that fifty thousand lives would be saved every year by taking statins, it would be considerably more accurate to state that if ten million people (at very high risk of heart disease) took a statin for a year they would all live – on average – two days longer. And if all ten million took a statin for two hundred years, they would all live – on average – an extra year.

If we assume that most people would take a statin for thirty years, maximum, this would lead to an average increase in lifespan of approximately two months. Which doesn't sound quite as dramatic as saving fifty thousand lives a year, or a thousand a week – or however else you choose to hype up your figures. But there you go, it happens to be considerably more accurate.

Also remember that this benefit would only be seen in men with pre-existing heart disease. Women and men without pre-existing heart disease would live not a day longer. They would just have the dubious pleasure of thirty years of paying for drugs, worry and side effects.

Perhaps you think that I am also manipulating statistics in a way to make my point. Maybe. But an increase in average survival time is how all results are presented in cancer trials. This is one reason why, I think, cancer trials tend to look rather unimpressive when stacked up against the highly dramatic 'life-saving' cardiovascular studies*.

Anyway, moving back to the main point of this section. In secondary prevention studies (in men) it seems that statins do lower cardiovascular mortality, and by enough to wipe out any increase in other causes of death. But do they do it by lowering LDL levels, or do they do it through other mechanisms?

This is not, actually, an easy question to answer with absolute certainty. Maybe by now you feel it doesn't much matter any more – given that you have just been made aware of the minute benefits that statins offer, even in the highest risk groups. However, I think it is important to look at this issue for two reasons:

- If I can prove that statins do not work by lowering LDL levels, then the entire 'cholesterol hypothesis' totally disintegrates.
- Currently, the combined might of the pharmaceutical industry plus opinion leaders are pressing hard for ever-greater LDL lowering and they are deliberately blurring the distinction between primary and secondary prevention. I think that this must be resisted, as it will lead to more and more people being put on very high doses of very potent statins, which would be a complete disaster.

But where to start? Where indeed.

When the first statin trials came out, it's true that they did seem to provide definitive proof that statins worked by lowering LDL levels. After all, they did exactly what they were supposed to: lower LDL and protect against CHD.

But it didn't take long before whole series of anomalies emerged which suggested that statins might be working through other mechanisms rather than by LDL lowering. The non-lipid actions are

---

* Actually, it is an increase in 'median' survival that is used. However, while the difference between average and median can be technically important, in most cases the two things are virtually the same. The reason why 'median' increase in survival is not used in cardiology is that it would take a hell of a long time for 50 per cent of the people to die. Not unfortunately usually a problem in cancer trials.

now bundled under the heading 'pleiotropic' effects (see Glossary for full explanation of this term).

And so a debate has emerged. A rather one-sided debate, given the scale of the respective budgets supporting either faction. But it is a debate nonetheless. Do statins protect by lowering LDL, or in other ways?

In the 'statins don't work by lowering LDL levels' corner are the following facts. This is only a small selection:

- Statins protect against dying of heart failure, despite the fact that a high LDL level is associated with increased survival in this condition.
- The beneficial effects of statins have been seen within weeks, days, even hours of taking a statin. And this finding does not remotely fit with the hypothesis that raised LDL creates gradual plaque build-up over years and years[9].
- Statins protect against strokes, but a raised cholesterol level is not a risk factor for stroke.
- Statins provide the same degree of protection no matter if the LDL level is high, average, or low (HPS study).
- Some studies, such as CARE, showed that the greatest degrees of LDL lowering were associated with a rise in deaths from heart disease.

While some of us may say, 'Who cares? If they work, they work,' if you have spent a lifetime, and built your glittering reputation, 'proving' that raised LDL causes heart disease, you are not going to allow facts like these to remain standing.

Equally, if you are trying to sell a statin-based drug entirely on the awesome power of its LDL-lowering properties, you are not going to take kindly to an alternative explanation jamming up the works. And so, a series of studies were set up designed to prove, for good and all, that the more you lower LDL, the greater the protection against heart disease.

9 In 4S, no benefits were seen until 18 months. Which is very odd, considering that all other trials have shown much more rapid effects. What were Mereck doing?

The major studies were PROVE-IT, TNT, A to Z, REVERSAL, ASTEROID and IDEAL. No, there will not be a test at the end of this chapter to remember which was which, or what was what. Or which proved what, why or how. After all, even the acronyms themselves are impossible to remember. And a bit bonkers too – witness ASTEROID (**A S**tudy **T**o **E**valuate the effect of **R**osuvastatin **O**n **I**ntravascular Ultrasound-**D**erived Coronary Atheroma Burden). Wheee!

Let's look firstly at the IDEAL study – the biggest. After it ended, Scott Grundy – who, it must be said, is a statinoholic – wrote an article entitled 'The clinical implications of IDEAL: in the context of Recent Intensive Statin Therapy Trials' for Medscape. I quote:

> *We now have very clear evidence that patients with established CAD [heart disease] will benefit from intensive LDL-Cholesterol [LDL-C]- lowering therapy.*

In short, case closed: statins work by lowering LDL levels, now will you all please shut up? This, I have to say, I find an extremely interesting interpretation, given the results themselves.

The IDEAL study – it should be pointed out – was very big. Twice the size of 4S, with 8,888 patients, no less. Patients were either put on 20mg or 40mg of simvastatin (the doses used in 4S), or 80mg of atorvastatin (Lipitor). LDL was lowered by 33 per cent in the simvastatin group and 42 per cent in the atorvastatin group. The result: *'No statistically significant differences were seen in all-cause mortality, cardiovascular mortality, or non-cardiovascular mortality.'* (In fact, cardiovascular mortality was very slightly higher in the atorvastatin group.) Despite this, according to the study's author, we now have very clear evidence that patients with established heart disease will benefit from more intensive LDL/cholesterol lowering… This is an interpretation that flatly contradicts the results of the study itself. Although, to be perfectly frank, I see a trend of analysis of trials that bears no relation to my interpretation of these trials.

Maybe he misunderstood the key findings that *'No statistically* significant differences were seen in all-cause mortality, cardiovascular mortality, or non-cardiovascular mortality'? Maybe this wasn't quite clear cut enough for him? Perhaps, he just missed the word 'No' at the start of the sentence? Easy to do that, I find.

And what of ASTEROID? You may remember that this study was hyped to the very skies, appearing as a major news item on the BBC, no less, under the headlines 'Drug can reverse heart disease' – with pretty pictures of disappearing plaques, just to make the point.

Not everyone was that impressed. Dr Graham Jackson, a UK cardiologist, wrote an editorial on the matter in the *International Journal of Clinical Practice*. I quote a selection of his views on ASTEROID:

> *As a marketing exercise it was brilliant. As an educational exercise it exploited sensationalism. And as a scientific exercise it was another own goal for the pharmaceutical industry (AstraZeneca provided a press release which went largely uncriticised and could be seen as part of a direct-to-the-public advertising campaign)... So what was so stunning about ASTEROID? Nothing really...*

The study was headed by Dr Steven Nissen. Of the ASTEROID trial itself, Dr Nissen stated that he had never seen regression of atherosclerotic plaques in his entire career before this. This sounds similar to his reaction to the ApoA-1 Milano trial two years previously: *'We really didn't think it was going to work,'* Nissen told WebMD. *'Nobody was more shocked than I was when the statisticians handed me the data... It is unprecedented. Nobody has even seen this kind of plaque regression. It really is an epiphany.'* In relation to another intensive LDL-lowering trial that he was in charge of, the REVERSAL trial:

> *'The results were striking,' Dr Nissen said, 'demonstrating a complete halting of coronary disease progression in the atorvastatin-treated patients and continued progression of disease in the pravastatin-treated group.'*

Dr Steven Nissen, it should be mentioned, was also the lead investigator in the most positive study on intensive LDL lowering that measured clinical end-points, rather than measuring plaque size with an ultrasound probe. It was called Treating to New Targets (TNT).

They say that lightning never strikes twice in the same place. Yet there have only been four major studies on intensive LDL lowering that have been positive, and Steve Nissen has been in charge of three of them. In fact, if you removed the Steven Nissen-controlled trials, the evidence on intensive LDL lowering would be almost entirely negative.

The only major positive study not run by Steven Nissen was PROVE-IT. Ironically, this study was set up by Bristol-Myers Squibb to prove that intensive LDL lowering had no added benefit to moderate LDL lowering. It seemed the ultimate own goal, as it appeared to end up proving the opposite. But did it?

Firstly, the bare bones of the trial itself. In PROVE-IT, the investigators took 4,162 patients who had been in hospital following an MI, or unstable angina (almost, but not quite an MI). They then split the group in half and gave one half pravastatin (made by Bristol-Myers Squibb), and the other half a much higher dose of atorvastatin (made by Pfizer). As expected, LDL level, or 'bad cholesterol' level, was reduced to a greater extent in the atorvastatin group.

- LDL in the treated pravastatin group: average 95 mg/dl (range 79–113)
- LDL in the treated atorvastatin group: average 62 mg/dl (range 50–79)

In short, in the atorvastatin group there was a 32 per cent greater reduction in LDL levels, and there was also a 16 per cent greater reduction in – well – almost everything you can think of: all-cause mortality, MI, unstable angina, hospital readmission, interventional procedures – you name it. It was all quite wonderful. In absolute terms, a somewhat less wonderful 0.5 per cent reduction in overall mortality per year.

My interpretation? Actually, I don't have one. You see, the researchers gave two different groups of patients two different doses of two different drugs. They then decided that all benefits seen were due to greater LDL lowering. How can they draw this conclusion? The answer is that they cannot. It's impossible to do so, unless you know that the two drugs are absolutely identical in all of their actions, other than the impact they have on LDL lowering.

If, for example, atorvastatin has non-LDL lowering benefits on CHD that pravastatin does not, this would be the reason for the difference. But how can anyone know. This has never been tested.

Ironically, the possibility that atorvastatin is better at preventing CHD than pravastatin, no matter what the LDL level, is supported by Dr Steven Nissen. In the REVERSAL study, which also used low dose pravastatin and high dose atorvastatin, he found the following:

> Surprisingly, despite attaining a low LDL level on pravastatin, these patients showed highly significant progression for percent atheroma volume and percent obstructive volume... At any LDL level, progression was less on atorvastatin than on pravastatin. When I started this study, I believed that any reduction in progression would just be due to lower LDL levels, but now I'm not so sure. This analysis suggests that it may be more than just LDL it seems to be the drug as well... Yes, this is a post-hoc analysis and should be considered hypothesis generating, but I would say it is a robust finding.

Goodness me, of all people.

This finding actually highlights the hopeless weakness at the centre of all the intensive LDL-lowering trials. They have almost all used different doses of different drugs. This is not a scientific technique that I would recommend if you ever want to actually prove anything, ever.

Even if they had used different doses of the same drug, you would not be able to say that it is the LDL lowering that created any benefit. It could have been another dose-dependent 'direct' drug effect that you haven't even measured, or don't even know exists.

Having said this, there has been one, and only one, major study done in which different doses of the same statin were used – the A to Z trial, using simvastatin. Guess what? Despite major differences in the LDL levels attained, there were no benefits seen from taking the higher dose of simvastatin on cardiovascular – or overall – mortality. This was despite the fact that the 'low-dose' group weren't actually given a statin for the first four months of the study. Bonkers.

Frankly, the intensive LDL-lowering studies have not actually proved anything at all – except, perhaps, that simvastatin and atorvastatin are superior in reducing the risk of CHD than pravastatin for – as yet – unknown reasons. And anyone who argues differently needs to be given a copy of *How to do Scientific Studies – for Five-Year-Olds*.

Rule one: If you have more than one uncontrolled variable in your study you can't prove anything.

Rule two: If you think you have proved something in a study with more than one uncontrolled variable, Rule one shall apply.

Summary
At this point I shall attempt to draw all the strands on the use of statins together. First the positive data:

- If you are a man with pre-existing heart disease, statins reduce your risk of dying of anything by a maximum of 0.66 per cent per year. (This figure is based on the most positive data from the most positive study – 4S. Study run by Merck, primary data analysis carried out by Merck employee.)
- If you are a man without pre-existing heart disease, statins can reduce your risk of dying of cardiovascular disease – by a small amount.
- If you are a woman at very high risk of heart disease, statins reduce the risk of dying of cardiovascular disease (that is, strokes and heart disease).

Then the less positive data:

- If you are a woman, no matter what your level of risk, statins will not increase your life expectancy by one day. Deaths from cardiovascular disease reduced; deaths from other causes increased.
- If you are a man without heart disease, statins will not increase your life expectancy by one day.

Then the negative data:

- Statins, cholesterol tests and GP appointments and screening are costing the NHS alone billions of pounds a year.
- Statins cause muscle pains and muscle weakness in up to 20 per cent of people who take them.
- Statins cause rhabdomyolysis, which can be fatal.
- One type of statin, simvastatin, over a period of six years, caused 416 deaths in the USA alone.
- Statins cause polyneuropathy.
- Statins cause memory loss, depression, confusion, irritability and dizziness.
- Stains cause major birth defects.

Finally, a couple of worrying, though unproved, possibilities:

- Statins may increase cancer risk.
- Statins may cause heart failure.

It is also, as yet, not remotely proven that statins protect against heart disease by lowering LDL levels. The current hyping of the intensive LDL-lowering trials has been driven purely by the pharmaceutical industry. They claim to have proved beyond doubt that the more the LDL is lowered, the greater the protection against heart disease, and they have tried to use this 'fact' to press for ever-greater cholesterol lowering in the entire population.

CHAPTER 9

WHAT CAUSES HEART DISEASE?

My interest in heart disease was first piqued, many moons ago, by the knowledge that the French had a very low rate of heart disease, despite having the entire raft of conventional risk factors. Over the years, I have found far more outstanding paradoxes than the French, but at that time they stuck out like a sore thumb, a mute reproach to the conventional theories about heart disease. A reproach that people have continually tried, and failed, to explain.

To be frank, I found the mainstream excuses about the protective effects of eating garlic, drinking red wine and lightly cooking their vegetables to be utter bunk. It was obvious that these factors had only emerged to keep the cholesterol hypothesis alive and sweep the French paradox under the carpet.

But what else, I thought, could explain the low rate of heart disease in France? As I'm from Scotland – where the heart disease rate at the time I became interested was the highest in the world – my mind turned to the way that the French eat, and the importance of food and eating, in their culture. In Scotland, eating is seen as somewhat akin to filling up your car with petrol. A waste of ten minutes, but it is something that has to be done before going out and getting 'pished' on a Saturday night.

As for cooking, my memory of a traditional Scots recipe is, as follows:

Step one: Place a three-pound lump of beef in a saucepan with a
carrot and an onion and boil for eight hours.

Step two: Eat with boiled potatoes.

And as everyone knows, the Scots love a fry-up. Even a fried-up
Mars bar:

Step one: Take a frozen Mars bar and cover in batter. Place in deep-fat
fryer for two minutes.
Step two: Eat with chips while walking home in the rain.

When I was growing up in Scotland, there used to be a substance
called zinc ointment – maybe there still is. If you have never heard of it,
thank the Lord. It was used as a cream substitute in things like
chocolate éclairs. The Scots felt that cream tasted far too delicious to
besmirch their puritanical souls. Therefore, it should be replaced with
an off-white substance of little taste, although such taste as it had was
distinctly bitter and unpleasant. I suspect it was constructed entirely
from E-numbers in a petrochemical plant.

A few years back, I took my wife to watch Dunfermline Athletic play
football. During the match, she made the extremely rash decision to
buy a mutton pie. I did warn her, but she wouldnae listen, she just
wouldnae. A mutton pie washed down with Bovril, no less. However, it
is the mutton pie itself that is a true specialité de la Scottish cuisine. A
pastry coating that the British Army has since discovered can prevent
uranium-depleted shells from piercing tank armour. And if you do
manage to get through this defensive barrier without breaking your
teeth, you will discover a small piece of gristle, surrounded by half a
pint of grey, liquid fat. The fat usually spurts out, covering all clothing
within a ten-foot radius, and it cannot be removed by any form of
washing powder yet created.

As a general observation, therefore, it can be said that food and
eating, are not given quite the same status in Scotland as in France. For

the French, food is a central part of life. Mealtimes are a major social occasion. People spend a long time buying food, preparing meals and then eating. In Scotland they don't, or at least they certainly didn't. This, to me, marked a very obvious difference between the two countries.

Could this attitude to food and eating somehow be the reason for the difference in heart-disease rates between the two countries? And if so, how? Was it something to do with being relaxed while trying to digest food, rather than shovelling it down as fast as possible?

With this thought in mind, I began what turned into a 25-year journey of discovery. It has to be said that I have taken many wrong turns along the way. There were several years when I thought that heart disease did not actually have a cause, or causes at all, so often did I find myself in another blind alleyway. Eventually, everything did come together in a way that makes sense and is actually supported by the facts. The primary cause of heart disease, I finally discovered, is... stress.

Well, hey, like haven't about ten million people been saying this for the last fifty years? Indeed they have. However, there is a major problem here, which is that the word 'stress' doesn't really mean anything at all. Or perhaps it means too many things. Or perhaps it just means different things to different people.

So how can anyone say that stress causes heart disease, when there is little agreement as to what stress actually means? It's a good question. In order to answer it, I have to attempt to define rather more clearly what I mean by stress.

WHAT IS STRESS?

I suppose many people think of stress as a form of time pressure. Busy, busy, busy, so much to do, so little time to do it. Others think of stress as a type of constant grinding worry, like money problems, or having an oppressive boss at work. Stress can also be seen as a transient state – for instance, moving house, or getting married, or even getting up on a Monday morning.

Many people believe that stress is good for us, and without it we would just lounge about doing nothing at all – certainly true in my case. This lack of any clear definition, or even agreement about fundamental principles, such as whether stress per se is healthy, or unhealthy, does make it tricky to measure it in any repeatable way. And without a measurement the medical profession tends to lose interest rapidly.

With a cholesterol test, you know exactly what you're getting. It's 5.9, or 6.2, or 3.8, or 2.79. Once you have your figure, you can then give drugs and watch the figure change in front of your very eyes. Then you can draw graphs, do an audit, write papers… and all sorts of things. Proper science, no less. The sort that gets published in proper journals and leads to proper promotions.

But with things like stress, no such measurements exist. We are in the world of the subjective experience, where we have to rely on personal testimony and suchlike. It is not a place where many medical researchers like to venture.

An Eastern Tale
(As told to me)

A stranger was passing through a village one day when he spotted a wise man scrabbling about in the dust. 'What are you doing?' asked the stranger. 'I am looking for my key,' replied the wise man. 'I shall help,' the stranger exclaimed, and immediately set about the search. He looked under leaves, he sifted in the dust, he looked everywhere. After about two hours there was still no sign of the key. 'Are you sure you lost it out here?' the by now very dusty and thirsty stranger asked. 'Oh, no,' the wise man replied. 'I lost it in my house.' Understandably, the stranger was somewhat irritated. 'Then why are we looking out here?' he demanded. The wise man smiled. 'Because,' he said 'out here the light is so much better for looking.'

I have to admit that I too, enjoy looking where the light is so much better. But sometimes you have to bite the bullet and accept that this doesn't actually happen to be where the answers lie. And with stress, and heart disease, you must search in a world where some of the answers cannot be directly seen. You can only know they are there by the effects that they have on things around them.

Just to give one example, from a study published in the BMJ in 2001 entitled 'The Hound of the Baskervilles effect: natural experiment on the influence of psychological stress on timing of death':

In Mandarin, Cantonese, and Japanese, the words 'death' and 'four' are pronounced nearly identically, and consequently the number 4 evokes discomfort and apprehension in many Chinese and Japanese people. Because of this, the number 4 is avoided in floor and room numbers in some Chinese and Japanese hospitals, and in some Chinese and Japanese restaurant telephone numbers. In addition, the mainland Chinese airforce avoids the number 4, but uses other numbers, to designate its military aircraft, apparently because of the superstitious association between 'four' and 'death'.

The study by Phillips and his co-authors finds that cardiac deaths peak on the fourth of the month for Americans of Chinese and Japanese descent, and that this pattern is not seen among whites. The study used computerized US death certificates to examine more than 200,000 Chinese and Japanese deaths, and 47,000,000 white deaths, from 1973 to 1998.

On one hand we have a real and scientifically measurable effect, which is that Chinese and Japanese die more often on the fourth day of the month – and you can't argue with that, it's a fact. On the other hand, we have something much more difficult to deal with, which is that the reason for this increased risk of death appears to be that the Chinese and Japanese consider the number four to be unlucky.

But has anyone worked out how to measure the physiological effect of 'unluckiness'? Can we invent a drug to protect against the damage cause by the number four? I tend to doubt it. Yet the deadly effect of 'four' exists, nonetheless.

So what do we do? Simply ignore this finding, because it is considered virtually impossible to analyse in the reductionist way so beloved of medical science? Or do we bite the bullet and accept that, for some people, the number four can cause deadly stress? Even if we must also accept that it is very tricky to get a handle on what it is about this number that creates stress? I suggest the latter.

However, the mainstream has tended to the former approach, i.e. ignoring. Just to give one example of this tendency, a huge study was carried out in 52 countries looking at 29,000 people in order to establish the similarities, or differences, between risk factors across a wide range of different populations. This was the INTERHEART study.[10]

As part of INTERHEART, they measured psychosocial stress – hallelujah! Annika Rosengren, Professor of Cardiology at Goteborg University, Sweden – who led the stress aspect of the research – noted that people's psychosocial wellbeing, judged by simple measures, was significant:

> 'Collectively these [measures] were responsible for about one third of the risk of the population studies,' she said. 'Persistent severe stress makes it two and a half times more likely that an individual will have a heart attack compared with someone who is not stressed.' She said stress and depression together increased the risk threefold.
>
> 'The public thinks stress is very important in their heart attack. My patients often say they think it was due to stress, but previous studies have shown contrary effects of stress. But the INTERHEART study shows definitively that stress is one of the most important factors in heart attack in all ethnic groups and in all countries.'
>
> http://www.telegraph.co.uk/news/main.jhtml?xml=/news/2004/ 09/02/wstres02.xml&sSheet=/portal/2004/09/02/ixportal.html

10 Yusuf S, Hawken S, Ounpuu S, on behalf of the INTERHEART Study Investigators. 'Effect of potentially modifiable risk factors associated with myocardial infarction in 52 countries (the INTERHEART study): case-control study'. *The Lancet*, 2004; 364:937–952.

Most interesting, and surely something worth pursuing further? However, the mainstream response to this was best encapsulated, in the same article, by Professor Sir Charles George, Medical Director of the British Heart Foundation. He did say that the results 'suggested' that stress might have more of a role as a cause of heart attacks than many people had previously thought. (*Don't you just love the use of that word 'suggested'?*) However, he went on to caution that the findings were the result of 'self-reported' stress that had not been confirmed by chemical measures – of hormones in saliva, for example. In short, you didn't really measure it in the approved scientific manner, therefore it doesn't really exist. In such a casually dismissive fashion is the evidence about perceived stress swept under the carpet, time and time again.

Of course, stress is not a simple concept, and measuring it is even more difficult. However, if you are willing to accept proof, and facts, that are less rigid than $p < 0.005$ (CI 0.63 – 84), then good. After all, as Albert Einstein was wont to say:

> Not everything that can be measured, matters, and not everything that matters can be measured.
> [One of several different versions of this saying attributed to him.]

This does not mean that I am simply going to claim that stress is the main cause of heart disease and leave it at that. Indeed, I intend to use a great deal of evidence to make the case for – or should that be against – stress. Just because you can't accurately measure everything does not mean that you should give up, or try to use good scientific research wherever possible.

At this point, therefore, having thrown enough caveats into the air to sink a battleship, I will take the plunge and attempt to show you exactly how stress causes heart disease. Before I can do this, though, I have to dismantle stress into its component parts.

Firstly, we'll need to separate out the things that cause stress – the 'stressors' – from the 'stress response', i.e. the physiological effects that stressors create. Of course, not all stressors will create a stress response. For example, the number four will have no effect on most people in the West-whereas the number thirteen might.

After separating cause and effect, a further split is necessary because there are two basic stress responses: healthy and unhealthy. As a further subdivision, I need to make the distinction between the two types of stressor: physical and psychological.

To try and make this a bit clearer, I have created a list of the type of stressors I am talking about, and the likely effects that they have.

1: Examples of physical stressors that create a healthy response:

- Exercise
- Competitive sport
- Massage
- Sauna
- Moderate alcohol consumption
- Singing
- Bungee jumping
- Rock climbing
- Roller-coaster rides

2: Examples of psychological stressors that create a healthy stress response:

- Your football team winning
- Passing an exam
- Clinching a successful business deal
- Organising an enjoyable social evening
- A tight sales deadline – but not too tight
- Giving a well-received lecture
- A busy shift in Accident and Emergency with no one dying
- Being Prime Minister

3: Examples of physical stressors that create an unhealthy stress response:

- Excessive, intense, forced exercise in adverse conditions, e.g. working deep below the ground in a coal mine in Russia
- Extreme environmental change/rapid alteration in temperature
- Being a fighter-jet pilot
- Rheumatoid arthritis
- Cocaine use
- Smoking
- Eating under pressure
- Major trauma/surgery
- Spinal cord injury
- Steroid use
- Disease of the hormonal system
   - Cushing's disease (too much cortisol)
   - Phaechromocytoma (too much adrenaline)
   - Diabetes (too much blood sugar)
   - Acromegaly (too much growth hormone)

4: Examples of psychological stressors that create an unhealthy stress response:

- Bullying boss
- Suffering racism
- Being 'dislocated' from the surrounding population/culture
- Money worries, long-term debt
- Low status in social hierarchy
- Poor social network
- Non-supportive, unloving or abusive spouse
- Football team losing
- Getting caught in an earthquake (though this is a physical stressor too)
- Getting up on Monday morning
- Forced emigration/social dislocation
- The number four

These are not full lists, by any manner of means – and not all of the things on these lists will create the same response in all people. But I hope that it gives you a clearer idea of the types of 'stressors' that I am talking about. My next trick is to explain exactly how an unhealthy stress response (whatever causes it) goes on to cause heart disease.

HOW AN UNHEALTHY STRESS RESPONSE CAUSES HEART DISEASE

In order to explain how this happens, I need to introduce you to the neurohormonal system. This hugely complex system consists of two basic parts: the 'hormonal' part and the 'nervous system' part. While I have provisionally called this the 'stress system', the term is actually horribly inaccurate. Because the system involved in stress is precisely the same system that is involved in relaxation – only in reverse.

In fact, for every hormone in the neurohormonal system that fires you up, there is another one that calms you down; and for every set of nerve fibres that revs you up, there is another network that relaxes you. Eastern philosophy would call this whole shebang Yin and Yang, internal balance, which is a pretty good way of looking at it. Because if the neurohormonal system gets seriously out of balance, you are likely to suffer catastrophic metabolic problems, then heart disease... then cancer, then diabetes, then... well, too much for me to cover in one book.

The hormones involved on the 'stress' side include adrenaline, cortisol, growth hormone and glucagon. On the 'relaxation' side, for the purposes of this discussion, I shall concentrate on insulin.

Release of stress hormones is controlled by the hypothalamus and pituitary gland acting in unison. Under a stressful situation – for example, a man pointing a gun at you – the hypothalamus sends alarm messages to the pituitary gland, which then fires off hormonal messengers to the adrenal glands to get them to release adrenaline and cortisol, among other things.

This 'three-part' hormonal system, consisting of the hypothalamus, pituitary gland and adrenal glands, is often referred to as the

Hypothalamic-Pituitary-Adrenal axis, or the HPA-axis for short. The HPA-axis is intimately connected to, and intertwined with, the unconscious or 'autonomic' nervous system. The autonomic nervous system has two basic divisions: the sympathetic and the parasympathetic systems. Neither of these divisions is under your conscious control – unless you are a Zen master, or something of the sort.

Fig. 29 The parasympathetic and sympathetic nervous systems

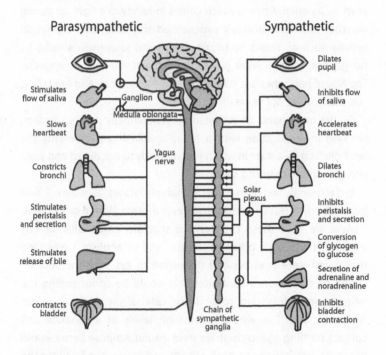

Parasympathetic

Sympathetic

Stimulates flow of saliva

Ganglion

Medulla oblongata

Slows heartbeat

Yagus nerve

Constricts bronchi

Solar plexus

Stimulates peristalsis and secretion

Stimulates release of bile

contratcts bladder

Chain of sympathetic ganglia

Dilates pupil

Inhibits flow of saliva

Accelerates heartbeat

Dilates bronchi

Inhibits peristalsis and secretion

Conversion of glycogen to glucose

Secretion of adrenaline and noradrenaline

Inhibits bladder contraction

The sympathetic nervous system has a wide range of actions. These include speeding up your heart rate, reducing saliva production and redirecting blood supply to your muscles. It also stimulates the liver to release glucose, thus pushing up blood-sugar levels, and triggers the release of various blood-clotting factors. These are the sort of things you need when physical danger threatens, which is why this whole process is sometimes called the 'fight or flight' response.

On the other hand the parasympathic nervous system has directly opposing actions. It slows your heart, stimulates insulin production and the release of bile. It also increases the flow of saliva, and directs blood to the guts to aid digestion.

Another way to look at this is to say that an activated sympathetic nervous system – working in conjunction with raised 'stress' hormones – represents the 'catabolic' state, a state in which your body is ready to burn up its energy stores, which comes in handy in a fight, or during exercise. You have probably experienced this state after a physical activity such as tennis or squash, when you know you should be hungry but find that when you sit down to eat you have no appetite. The 'stress' hormones are still ruling your metabolism, and are telling you that you are not yet ready to eat.

On the other hand, an activated parasympathetic nervous system, working in conjunction with a raised insulin level, represents the 'anabolic' state – a state in which you are ready to eat, digest and store energy – and then have a siesta.

In fact, analysing these two metabolic 'states' is where I first began in my quest to understand heart disease. Within our bodies, I knew, we have these two systems that are, essentially, directly antagonistic to each other. Anabolism and catabolism. I reasoned that if you were stressed, and then tried to eat, your metabolism would be thrown into confusion. You would be commanding the neurohormonal system to activate catabolism and anabolism simultaneously. This would mean high levels of adrenaline and cortisol, battling against high levels of insulin. Adipose tissue would be under instructions to both absorb and pump out fats into the bloodstream. At the same time, the liver would be trying to store, and release, glucose.

With food inside them, your guts would be automatically switched to 'absorption'. But the sympathetic system would be fighting to direct blood away from the guts to the muscles. Wherever you looked, a fight for metabolic supremacy would be going on. Perhaps the most important battle would be for control of blood-sugar levels, a battle ending up with 'spikes' of blood sugar – as insulin tried, and most likely failed, to overcome the effects of the stress hormones surging about in the bloodstream.

In short, I thought that eating under stress was likely to be pretty damned unhealthy. Equally, taking time over meals, and relaxing while doing so, was likely to be pretty damned healthy. Could this be the reason for the high rate of heart disease in Scotland, and the low rate of heart disease in France? Possibly, probably… it almost certainly represents part of the answer.

More on that later. Now it is time to look at what happens when the 'stress system' breaks down. Actually, from now on, I am going to refer to a breakdown of the stress system as a 'dysfunctional HPA-axis'. Sorry about using this jargon, but it is much more accurate and useful. It also moves the discussion away from the slightly woolly concept of stress, to something that can be measured, i.e. HPA-axis function. (Normally this is done by measuring cortisol levels.)

Causes of a dysfunctional HPA-axis

Probably the most dramatic dysfunction of the HPA-axis occurs when a tumour develops in the pituitary gland, which then proceeds to pump out far too much in the way of stress hormones. Several types of these tumours can develop. A tumour producing too much growth hormone can lead to gigantism and acromegaly; a tumour producing too much adrenaline can cause a condition known as phaeochromocytoma, etc.

However, I am only going to focus on one type: a tumour in the pituitary gland that pumps out too much ACTH (corticotropin). ACTH is a 'precursor' hormone which, in turn, stimulates cortisol secretion from the adrenal glands. So, a tumour in the pituitary gland, (secreting too much ACTH) effectively increases blood cortisol levels. This condition is known as Cushing's disease.

Cushing's disease, in turn, has a wide range of different effects –

which are a direct result of the many actions that cortisol has around the body. For example, cortisol:

- Triggers the liver to release its stores of glucose.
- Stimulates the breakdown of triglyceride stores in adipose tissue, leading to an increase in free fatty acids (FFAs) in the blood. Triglyceride breakdown also releases glycerol, which travels directly to the liver, where it is converted to glucose.
- Activates breakdown of muscle protein into amino acids. (The amino acids then travel to the liver, where they are converted into glucose.)
- Acts as a direct antagonist to the actions of insulin at most sites in the body.

As you might expect, therefore, people with too much cortisol surging about in the system have high blood-sugar levels and a high degree of what is known as 'insulin resistance'. In fact, most people with Cushing's disease develop diabetes.

Another thing that happens to people with Cushing's disease is that they lose muscle bulk – due to the breakdown of muscle proteins. There is also a redistribution of fat from the periphery (arms and legs) to the trunk, or abdomen. Sometimes this redistribution can be so extreme that it leads to a condition known as 'buffalo' hump.

The reason why this happens is because you have two very different types of fat in your body: subcutaneous and visceral. Subcutaneous fat sits just underneath the skin and is found all over the place: arms, legs, neck, even fingers. Sumo wrestlers have lots of this type of fat, and they work hard to build it up. How they do this is a fascinating topic. (Well, at least I find it fascinating, but this is not time to get sidetracked.)

Visceral fat, on the other hand, is mainly found around the organs in your abdomen. It is the type of fat that builds up in those who develop the classic 'beer belly'. While both types of adipose tissue can each store, and then release, fat, that is the beginning and end of any similarity. From a metabolic perspective, they are as different as different can be. They are to all intents and purposes different organs. One is fat, the other is 'anti-fat'.

I shall tiptoe around this area because it is both enormous, and enormously complex, and I do not want to get bogged down. Suffice to say, for the sake of this discussion, that cortisol stimulates subcutaneous adipose tissue to release fat, thus making it shrink in size. On the other hand, cortisol stimulates visceral fat to do the exact opposite, i.e. absorb and store fats, leading to an increase in visceral fat mass (This is a horrible oversimplification, but for the sake of this argument it will do.)

There is another reason for bringing these two types of fat into the discussion at this point, which is that a build-up of visceral fat is now recognised as a major risk factor for heart disease. In fact, many people now believe that visceral fat is the primary underlying abnormality in heart disease, as it is thought to create a wide spectrum of metabolic abnormalities that are closely linked to heart disease. These abnormalities have been brought under the umbrella term 'Syndrome X.' Also known, among other things, as:

- Metabolic syndrome X
- Reaven's syndrome
- Metabolic syndrome
- Insulin resistance syndrome

Whatever you choose to call it (and please will someone make up their minds!), to my mind the current thinking is bonkers. Visceral fat doesn't build up all by itself, just for the hell of it, before going on to create Syndrome X. Something has to cause the build-up of visceral fat in the first place. To argue otherwise is to end up in the mad genetics/magic argument again: 'Visceral fact accumulation just, sort of, happens. We don't know why, so it must be due to genetic susceptibility.' (Listen, guys, it doesn't just happen. It is caused by HPA-axis dysfunction and abnormal cortisol levels. Hellooo! have a look at Cushing's disease!)

Anyway, in addition to its effects on raising glucose and insulin levels, and its impact on muscle and fat distribution, a high cortisol level also causes the following abnormalities:

- Raised VLDL level
- Low HDL level
- Raised LDL level
- Raised blood pressure
- Raised fibrinogen levels (clotting factor)
- Raised PAI-1 level (clotting factor)
- Raised Von Willibrand level (clotting factor)
- Raised Lp(a) level (clotting factor)

Does anything seem familiar about this list? If not, it will.

To round off this topic, I should probably mention that people with Cushing's disease have accelerated atherosclerotic plaque growth, and a gigantically increased risk of heart disease.

Strongly reinforcing the fact that it is the raised cortisol level itself that is causing the damage – rather than some other factor – is the evidence from people who take steroids. Steroids, as mentioned before, are among the most widely prescribed of all medications. They are also called 'corticosteroids', because the basic building block of all steroids is cortisol. What this means is that when you take a steroid you are, effectively, giving yourself Cushing's disease.

Why would anyone want to do this? Well, one effect of cortisol that I haven't mentioned so far is that it greatly inhibits the immune system. I haven't the faintest idea why cortisol does this. However, because it does, it is used to treat diseases when you want to shut down an overactive immune response. Such 'autoimmune' diseases include rheumatoid arthritis, asthma, eczema and ulcerative colitis. Steroids are also used after a transplant, as they prevent the body from rejecting the organ.

In situations like this, steroids are powerful and life-saving drugs. However, if you keep taking them for too long you will end up with the exact same set of abnormalities found in Cushing's disease: high blood-sugar and insulin levels, low HDL, high VLDL/ LDL, a whole range of blood-clotting factor abnormalities, and increased visceral fat deposition. In short, the works.

What's more, people who take steroids long term are at a greatly increased risk of dying of heart disease. Even fit, young, healthy people. And it can happen very fast. To give one example of the abuse of anabolic steroids (a form of cortisol/corticosteroid that has been altered to create muscle build-up, rather than break it down):

Anabolic steroids are frequently abused, thus increasing the risk of cardiovascular disease. We report on a young bodybuilder who presented with ventricular tachycardia as the first manifestation of severe underlying coronary heart disease. Coronary angiogram revealed severe stenotic lesions [narrowings] in the right coronary artery and the left descending coronary artery, and hypokinetic [hibernating] regions corresponding to posterolateral [the back and side] and anterior myocardial infarctions. This young patient had a history without any coronary risk factors, but with a 2-year abuse of the anabolic steroid stanazolol.

Mewis C Clin Cardiol, February 1996

Here is a young man with no classic risk factors for heart disease. Within two years of abusing steroids, however, he had developed severe occlusion in two major arteries in the heart, and he had also suffered two separate heart attacks (which he didn't actually know had happened). This looks like a fairly clear case of cause and effect to me.

Anyway, we have two different 'conditions' where cortisol levels are significantly raised: Cushing's disease and steroid use (or, rather, abuse). In both of them, exactly the same set of abnormalities develop, followed by heart disease. Clearly though, these two 'conditions' represent a very serious form of HPA-axis dysfunction indeed. You would almost certainly expect them to have a major destructive impact on the body. Equally clearly, not everyone who dies of heart disease has Cushing's disease, or takes steroids. So the next step is to show that other, less obviously severe forms of HPA-axis dysfunction also have the same destructive effect – through the same mechanisms. In order to do this, I want to look at three different initiators of HPA-axis dysfunction:

- Depression
- Smoking
- Spinal-cord injury

Depression first. It has long been known that people with depression are at a greatly increased risk of heart disease, but no one seems to be entirely certain why. However, when it has been studied it is clear that in depression you always find HPA-axis abnormalities.

> *There is compelling evidence for the involvement of hypothalamic-pituitary-adrenal [HPA-] axis abnormalities in depression. Growing evidence has suggested that the combined dexamethasone [DEX]/corticotropin-releasing hormone [CRH] test is highly sensitive to detect HPA axis abnormalities.*
>
> *Kunugi H, et al. Neuropsychopharmacology,*
> *January 2006; 3*

(I left in the stuff about the dexamthasone (DEX)/corticotrophin-releasing hormone (CRH) test for those who do like to see things properly measured, and refuse to believe in things that cannot be measured.)

In addition to the other metabolic problems, depression also leads to a build-up of visceral fat. I popped this observation in to make it clear that visceral-fat build-up is a result of underlying problems with the HPA-axis and raised cortisol levels – it doesn't happen by genetics. Or, indeed, magic.

> *We showed that depressive mood is associated with VAT [visceral adipose tissue], not with SAT [subcutaneous adipose tissue], in*

overweight premenopausal women. These findings may explain some of the association between depression and coronary heart disease. More studies are needed to elucidate the causal relationship.

Lee ES, et al, Obes Res, February 2005; 13

In fact, I think that depression is an almost perfect model to demonstrate that long-term dysfunctions of the HPA-axis – created purely by psychological stressors – works through exactly the same physical, and measurable, mechanisms as Cushing's disease to cause heart disease. Importantly, if you treat depression, the metabolic abnormalities often disappear – which represents reversibility of effect.

I didn't need to choose depression to show that psychological upset causes heart disease. I could have presented research on anxiety, or post-traumatic stress disorder, rather than depression. But I can assure you that research in all of these areas shows exactly the same thing. HPA-axis dysfunction, then metabolic abnormalities, then increased risk of death from heart disease. Once again, it is not a coincidence. This is a direct causal chain from HPA-axis upset to heart disease.

Smoking next. Although this may seem to be way out on a limb, it is not, because smoking actually works through exactly the same mechanisms as depression and Cushing's disease, although the effects are more likely due to repeated short-lived HPA-axis dysfunction, rather than chronic problems.

Two pieces of evidence. The first is taken from a study that looked at the effect of smoking a cigarette on cortisol and DHEA (dehydroepiandrosterone) levels (DHEA is a steroid hormone made in the adrenal glands in response to stress):

Cortisol and DHEA increased significantly within 20 min (P<0.05) and reached peak levels... within 60 and 30 min, respectively. Thus cigarette smoking produced nicotine dose-related effects on HPA hormones and subjective and cardiovascular measures.

Mendelson JH, et al, Neuropsychopharmacology,
September 2005; 30

The second study looked at the effects of smoking on ACTH and cortisol levels:

> *In the control group subjects, cigarette smoking induced a striking increase in the circulating concentrations of ACTH and cortisol, with peak responses 1.4 and 1.5 times higher than baseline at 20 and 30 min, respectively.*
> *Coiro V et al, Alcohol Clin Exp Res, September 1999; 23*

In addition to its effects on the HPA-axis, smoking also has a major impact on blood-clotting factors. Whether this is direct effect, or whether it is a result of HPA-axis activation, is not clear.

Finally, in this section, I wanted to mention spinal-cord injury. As with smoking, this may not initially seem to have anything to do with the HPA-axis dysfunction. However, the reality is that a spinal-cord injury impacts with massive force on the HPA-axis. This is because if you break vertebrae, and snap the spinal cord, you (usually) sever many of the sympathetic and parasympathetic nerves at the same time.

Unsurprisingly, this leads to enormous disruption in the entire neurohormonal system. The abnormalities found in spinal-cord injury are wide-ranging and, I regret to say, so complicated that I can't understand many of them myself. Indeed, most of the papers written in this area discuss hormones, and hormonal axes, that are beyond my ability to describe without tying myself in knots.

So I will use broad brush strokes here. If you want more information, you are perfectly welcome to go to www.pubmed.org and type in 'spinal-cord injury and/or cortisol levels and/or increased risk of CHD and/or increased visceral fat'. Here, you will find a whole series of papers outlining the same things – namely, that:

- Spinal-cord injury leads to severe HPA-axis dysfunction and raised cortisol levels.
- Patients with spinal-cord injury have low HDL levels (and other lipid abnormalities, e.g. raised VLDL levels).

- Patients with spinal-cord injury have sharply raised blood-clotting factors, including fibrinogen, Lp(a), and plasminogen activator inhibitor-1 (PAI-1).
- Spinal-cord injury leads to insulin resistance, up to and including frank diabetes.
- Spinal-cord injury patients develop visceral obesity.
- Spinal-cord injury patients are at a greatly increased risk of dying of heart disease.

Perhaps I am laying it on with a trowel here; perhaps not. By now, I hope you can see that HPA-axis dysfunction (and abnormal cortisol secretion) ties together a whole series of apparently disparate factors known to cause heart disease. To name but five, these include Cushing's disease, depression, use of steroids, smoking and spinal-cord injury. (Just try and find another way of linking these things to heart disease other than through HPA-axis dysfunction.)

In addition to this, HPA-axis dysfunction also explains where many of the 'classic' risk factors come from, e.g. low HDL, high VLDL/LDL, high blood pressure, diabetes, raised clotting factors and increased visceral-fat deposition. A dysfunctional HPA-axis is the underlying cause of these things.

Do these factors then go on to cause heart disease? Some of them may have a direct impact on heart disease – such as raised blood-clotting factors. Others are probably just signs of an underlying problem, e.g. low HDL levels. When so many things are tangled together, it is not that easy to say which causes what.

Anyway, as a sign-off to this section I want to return to the INTERHEART study. In this study, nine 'factors' were measured and found to have a close connection with heart disease. Six of them were associated with increased risk, and three of them were associated with reduced risk.

The six factors associated with increased risk of heart disease were:

- Smoking
- Diabetes

- Psychosocial stress
- High blood pressure
- Abdominal obesity (increased visceral fat)
- High ApoB/ApoA-1 ratio*

The authors of this paper treated each risk factor as acting in perfect isolation, having no relationship whatsoever to any other factors. However, I would like to point out that every single one of these six risk factors can be directly linked to a dysfunctional HPA-axis and raised/abnormal cortisol levels.

Two of them – smoking and psychosocial stress – are causes of HPA-axis dysfunction. Four of them result from HPA-axis dysfunction: high blood pressure, abdominal obesity, diabetes and dyslipidaemia.

As a quick aside, you may also have noted that, in this 52-country study, a raised LDL level, or raised cholesterol level, was not identified as a risk factor – something that seems to have passed everyone by. They fudged this finding horribly by using the strange concept of the ApoB/ApoA-1 ratio, and using the word 'dyslipidaemia' – suggesting the LDL was involved somewhere, but we know that it wasn't.

Finally, I would like to point out that the three factors in the INTERHEART study that protected against heart disease were:

- A high intake of fruit and vegetables
- Exercise
- Alcohol consumption

Two of these factors – exercise and alcohol consumption – have beneficial effects on the HPA-axis. You think I'm stretching it? Well, have a look at this quote from a study called 'The effect of a moderate level of white wine consumption on the hypothalamic-pituitary-adrenal axis before and after a meal':

* I have tried to find out what they meant by this ratio, but I cannot get an answer from the authors of the study. So, I have to assume this means a low HDL and raised VLDL and LDL level – as both of these lipoproteins have ApoB attached.

The results demonstrated a significant alcohol-induced decrease in salivary cortisol irrespective of nutritional status and a significant decrease in salivary DHEAS when alcohol is consumed... It was concluded that moderate white wine consumption may promote a transient alteration in the functioning of the HPA axis.

Pharmacol Biochem Behav, October–November 2001: 70

As for exercise, there is a huge mass of literature demonstrating very clearly that exercise is one of the best things you possibly do to maintain a healthy HPA-axis.

In fact, when you get down to it, the only factor in the INTERHEART study that cannot be related to the HPA-axis, at least not in any way that I know of, is the protective effect of eating fruit and vegetables.

So, while the authors stated that a mere one-third of the risk of heart disease could be due to psychosocial stress, if you look at the evidence in a different way it could be argued that the entire risk of heart disease is due to a dysfunctional HPA-axis – otherwise known as stress.

How do the abnormalities found with high cortisol levels
cause heart disease?

By now I hope to have convinced you that a whole range of different 'stressors' can upset the HPA-axis. Some operate over an extended period, some are transient but repeated, e.g. smoking. Some are physical; some psychological.

What I need to do now is make the final link in the chain. How do the metabolic abnormalities created go on to cause heart disease – or, to be more accurate, atherosclerotic plaque growth?

To answer this I need to return to the 'response to injury' hypothesis, first proposed by Carl Freiherr von Rokitansky more than 150 years ago. It's a hypothesis that has found support among many scientists over the years, and has an increasing following today – although it has to be said that, as with most hypotheses involved with heart disease, it has fragmented into a number of different versions. However, the basic concept is pretty straightforward, and I happen to think that it is correct.

In the 'response to injury' hypothesis, the first step in plaque formation is that a patch of endothelium (the thin, fragile, single-celled layer lining the arterial wall) becomes dysfunctional, damaged, or – more likely – is just plain stripped off.

When this happens, a section of the underlying arterial wall is exposed. This, in turn, acts as a very powerful stimulus to the clotting system to form a blood clot (or thrombus) to plug the gap. Once the thrombus has covered over the area of damage, the clotting process is brought to a halt. This is the basic 'response to injury'.

Then what happens? Well, for a moment, I would like you to have a think about what happens to your skin if you scratch or cut it. Blood escapes for a bit, then a clot/thrombus forms, which turns into a scab. After a while, the skin re-grows to seal up the scratch under the scab, and the scab falls off. If the same process were to happen in your arteries, then any blood clot that formed on a damaged bit of endothelium would eventually fall off, travel a bit further down the artery, and then jam solid once the artery narrowed. This would cause catastrophic problems – including, for example, strokes. Clearly, this is not a good thing. Therefore, blood clots forming on arteries cannot be allowed to fall off when the endothelial healing process is complete – unlike scabs on your skin.

In order to stop blood clots breaking off artery walls, and causing downstream havoc, they have to be drawn into the artery wall and then disposed of. How does this happen?

Answer: your bone marrow creates millions upon millions (upon billions, probably) of 'pre-endothelial' cells (also known as bone-marrow-derived vascular progenitor cells [VPCs]) that travel about in your bloodstream. When they see a breach in the endothelium, it's their job to cover it up.

Normally, however, a blood clot will have got there first, so these pre-endothelial cells stick to the surface of the blood clot, grow into full-blown endothelial cells, and cover over the damage with a new layer of endothelium. In this way, blood clots are, effectively, drawn into the arterial wall behind a new layer of endothelium. Usually they are then broken down, and removed, leaving no trace that they were ever there in the first place.

Now, you may be thinking, I hope, that this all makes perfect sense. But I have got to admit that the final part of this hypothesis about how arteries deal with blood clots is mine. I just kind of figured that it made sense. Having said this, virtually every other part of this hypothesis is known, and accepted. For example, everyone accepts that the endothelium can be damaged and everyone accepts that blood clots form over areas of damage. The only bit that is speculative is the idea that endothelial re-growth covers over thrombi, pulling them into the artery for disposal, rather than letting them break off and charge downstream. That said, frankly I don't know what everyone else thinks actually happens to thrombi that form on arterial walls, as there is no other version of events that makes sense. (I get the impression that most people haven't actually thought about this at all.)

I believe that this extended version of the 'response to injury' hypothesis is very strongly supported by some fascinating recent research done at Duke University in the USA:

> Scientists at Duke University Medical Center have discovered that a major problem with aging is an unexpected failure of the bone marrow to produce progenitor cells that are needed to repair and rejuvenate arteries exposed to such environmental risks as smoking or caloric abuse.
>
> The researchers demonstrated that an age-related loss of particular stem cells that continually repair blood vessel damage is critical to determining the onset and progression of atherosclerosis, which causes arteries to clog and become less elastic.
>
> http://dukemednews.org/news/article.php?id=6765&index=2

I would just ask the question: why would you have pre-endothelial cells circulating in your bloodstream if not to cover up areas of endothelial disruption? What else could they possibly be there for? Until a few years ago, no one even knew that these progenitor cells existed. Now they have been discovered – though, of course, if you think about it, they had to be there. Otherwise we would all be dead, as a damaged artery would never be able to repair itself.

The existence of progenitor cells also explains another issue that mainstream researchers have been grappling with for years. Namely (if you are still clinging to the cholesterol hypothesis), how can plaques form behind an intact endothelium, when LDL cannot penetrate intact endothelium? The answer is, of course, that plaques (which contain Lp(a) – a form of LDL – and LDL itself) start life as thrombi on top of damaged endothelium.

When new endothelial cells re-grow over the top of a thrombus they effectively draw it into the artery wall, along with Lp(a) and LDL. Puzzle solved: plaques don't actually form behind the endothelium at all. When they first form, that section of endothelium isn't actually there.

Moving on, if the processes that I have described up to now are 'healthy', what makes them become damaging? Or to put this another way, what causes a blood clot to remain stuck inside the artery wall, then grow into a big unstable plaque, instead of being disposed of by the repair systems (as I believe must happen to the majority of thrombi that form)?

The answer to this question is that plaques do not gradually grow by absorbing substances from the bloodstream, molecule by molecule, in some agonisingly slow diffusion-type process. They grow through repeated acute episodes of endothelial damage, followed by thrombus formation, all taking place on top of an existing plaque. In short, plaques grow in sudden, discrete episodes. And you don't need to take my word for this, because all the evidence I need for this version of events comes from the American Heart Association in their 'Scientific statement: a definition of advanced types of atherosclerotic lesions and a histological classification of atherosclerosis':

> *... 38% of persons with advanced lesions [plaques] had thrombi on the surface of the lesion. These thrombi ranged in size from minimal [microscopic] to grossly visible deposits, and some consisted of layers of different ages. Immunohistochemistry revealed wavy bandlike deposits related to fibrin [a key component of blood clots] within the advanced lesion of an additional 29% of persons. Because of their structure, these were thought to represent the remnants of old thrombi. Similar data were reported by other authors.*
>
> *The fissure and hematomas [a form of blood clot] that underlies thrombotic deposits in many cases may recur, and small thrombi reform many times. Repeated incorporation of small recurrent hematomas and thrombi into a lesion over months or years contributes to gradual narrowing of the arterial lumen.*

As this passage makes clear, repeated thrombus formation over plaques is what makes them get bigger. How else could you find fibrin, a key component of blood clots – and one that absolutely cannot pass through the endothelium – in distinct layers within plaques? How else could you find blood clots of different ages within plaques? You're right, you couldn't.

Further supporting the conjecture that thrombus formation is central to heart disease is the knowledge that the final event in heart disease is plaque rupture, with the formation of a very big blood clot on top of the plaque – big enough to completely block a coronary artery.

Almost all of this is accepted by the mainstream – with varying degrees of enthusiasm. What they will not accept is that the thing that gets the plaque started in the first place is endothelial damage, followed by formation of a blood clot. Even though this is exactly the same process that creates plaque enlargement and, eventually, fatal plaque rupture.

Why won't they accept this? Because it doesn't fit with the damnable cholesterol hypothesis. No hypothesis is allowed to exist that does not have a raised LDL at its heart. And the 'response to injury' hypothesis that I have outlined does not need LDL to make it work and also explains why a significant proportion of people who suffer heart attacks do not have a raised LDL. In fact, it explains everything.

Returning to the ground from my soapbox, I shall now tie a few things together:

- Plaques start life as small areas of damage to the endothelium, which are normally healed by the body's natural repair mechanisms – thrombus formation and endothelial re-growth.
- Plaques grow through repeated episodes of endothelial damage and blood-clot formation in the same spot.
- Plaques kill you when they 'rupture', creating a major blood clot that then blocks an important artery somewhere in the body.

Therefore, factors that cause accelerated plaque growth will be anything that has the capability either to damage the endothelium or cause more dangerous/bigger blood clots to form. Or both.

So what factors have been found to cause 'endothelial dysfunction'? They include:

- High blood-sugar levels, especially 'spikes' of blood sugar following a meal
- High insulin levels
- Acute mental stress
- Smoking
- Cocaine use
- Cortisol
- High levels of adrenaline

Okay so I have mixed up my factors a bit – some are mental disturbances and others are chemicals circulating in the blood – but you get the general drift. These are all factors that I have listed under the title 'unhealthy stressor', or else a downstream metabolic abnormality created by HPA-axis dysfunction.

I am not going to provide evidence to support this list. If you wish to check the facts for yourself, go to Google, or www.pubmed.org and type in 'endothelial dysfunction', followed by any one of these factors. You can then read the abstracts and papers for yourself. (I believe that this is a more honest form of referencing, rather than just picking the twenty or so papers that support my case, and failing to point out the ones that don't – though there aren't any of those anyway.)

Next, I think it is important to look at the factors that make the blood more ready to clot, and more ready to form big and difficult-to-shift blood clots. These are, somewhat unsurprisingly, blood-clotting factors, such as:

- Fibrinogen (Fibrinogen is a small strand of protein. When you stick hundreds of bits of fibrinogen together, it turns into a long, thin, very strong strand of fibrin. This binds blood clots together.)
- Lp(a)
- Plasminogen-activator-inhibitor-1 (PAI-1)
- Von-Willibrand factor
- VLDL (VLDL stimulates blood clots to form.)

I could actually go on giving you a list of clotting factors as long as your arm. Suffice to say that in study after study, you will find that raised blood-clotting factors are directly and consistently associated with an increased risk of heart disease, with no contradictory evidence in any study that I could find.

Although I could give you hundreds of studies supporting this statement, for the sake of brevity I will stick to one, from the New England Journal of Medicine, June 1995:

> In patients with angina pectoris, the levels of fibrinogen, von Willebrand factor antigen, and t-PA antigen are independent predictors of subsequent acute coronary syndromes. In addition, low fibrinogen concentrations characterize patients at low risk for coronary events despite increased serum cholesterol levels. Our data

are consistent with a pathogenetic role of impaired fibrinolysis [blood-clot break-down], endothelial-cell injury, and inflammatory activity in the progression of coronary artery disease.

The importance of blood clots in heart disease is also supported by the fact that virtually every drug that reduces the risk of dying of heart disease is, essentially, an anti-coagulant. For example:

- Aspirin – stops platelets becoming 'activated' and sticking together (activated platelets are critical to thrombus formation).
- Warfarin – reduces various clotting factors in the blood.
- Alcohol – stops platelets sticking together.
- Tissue plasminogen activator – breaks clots apart.
- Statins – have strong, dose-dependent, anti-coagulant activity.
- Streptokinase – a clot-buster.
- Clopidogrel – stops platelets sticking together (see aspirin).
- ACE-inhibitors (used to lower blood pressure) – ACE-inhibitors stimulate nitric oxide synthesis in endothelial cells. Nitric oxide is the most powerful anti-coagulant in the body.

On the other hand, drugs that increase the risk of blood clotting, such as Vioxx, greatly increase the risk of dying of heart disease.

The HPA-axis, response to injury model of heart disease
At this point, I believe it is now possible to put together a reasonably simple model of heart disease that leads from 'unhealthy stressor' to heart disease via HPA-axis dysfunction, raised cortisol levels and a series of metabolic abnormalities (see Fig. 30).

Of course, I am not the only person in the world to have recognised most, if not all, of these steps. In fact, a number of researchers are looking very closely at raised cortisol as the primary cause of heart disease.

The main reason for this sudden interest is the knowledge that the metabolic abnormalities of Cushing's disease are exactly the same as

Fig. 30 HPA-axis dysfunction 'response to injury' model

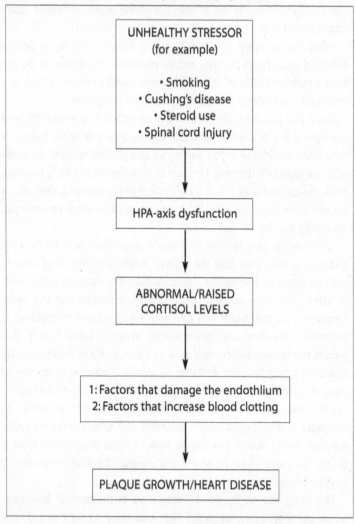

UNHEALTHY STRESSOR
(for example)

- Smoking
- Cushing's disease
- Steroid use
- Spinal cord injury

↓

HPA-axis dysfunction

↓

ABNORMAL/RAISED
CORTISOL LEVELS

↓

1: Factors that damage the endothlium
2: Factors that increase blood clotting

↓

PLAQUE GROWTH/HEART DISEASE

the metabolic abnormalities of Syndrome X. And Syndrome X is increasingly viewed as the number-one cause of heart disease – despite that fact that many in the mainstream refuse to recognise that it exists as a separate entity at all.

So what, you might ask, has stopped the model I presented above, or something very much like it, from becoming widely accepted (apart from the fact that it isn't the LDL hypothesis, of course)?

What has stopped it is the following simple fact. Many people suffering from heart disease, and/or metabolic Syndrome X, do not have a high cortisol level. In fact, it is often found to be low. Which, you might think, completely scuppers this model altogether.

But if you did think this, you would be wrong. The reason for your wrongness is that cortisol secretion usually peaks at about 8 a.m. – a time that coincides with you getting up and getting ready to do battle with the world for the next 16 hours or so. Following its early morning peak, the cortisol level falls during the rest of the morning, then rises a bit, then falls, then rises. This is all very much dependent on what you do during the day.

However, in people with HPA-axis dysfunction, very often what happens is that they lose the normal, healthy, flexible response to various stressors during the day, including the early morning peak. In effect, the HPA-axis 'burns out' and just pumps out the same amount of cortisol night and day, with no alteration in response. It becomes inflexible and non-variable. Which means that if you decide to measure the cortisol level at 8 a.m., or 9 a.m. (which are the standard times for such tests to be done), it can often be low in people with HPA-axis dysfunction – although not always, it depends on the degree of HPA-axis dysfunction. In reality, in order to diagnose HPA-axis dysfunction properly, you need to take repeated measurements during the day to look at what the cortisol level is doing. You also need to see if the normal 'healthy' response to stressors remains.

This brings me to the outstanding work of the late Per Bjorntorp. Some years ago, he recognised that you need to do more than a solitary cortisol measurement to diagnose HPA-axis dysfunction. He knew that the human body is a flexible and dynamic organism. Health, and healthy systems, are constantly adapting and reacting. When you lose flexibility and responsiveness, you die.

Perhaps the most spectacular example of this is heart-rate variability, i.e. the amount by which the heart rate alters from beat to beat. This is, possibly, the single most sensitive indicator of a healthy heart, and a loss of beat-to-beat variability is one of the most powerful single indicators of the risk of dying of heart disease.

Armed with such knowledge, Bjorntorp wasn't just looking for high, or low, levels of cortisol at 8 a.m. He was more interested in seeking a loss of HPA-axis flexibility, and 'burn-out' of the axis. To give one example of his work in his own, rather distinctly Swedish, words:

> *The conspicuous similarities between Cushing's disease and the Metabolic Syndrome X open up the possibility that hypercortisolaemia [high cortisol level] is involved in the latter. Salivary cortisol is possible to measure during undisturbed conditions including perceived stressful events during everyday life.*
>
> *Such measurements clearly show that normally regulated cortisol secretion is associated with excellent health in anthropometric, metabolic and hemodynamic variables. Upon perceived stress cortisol secretion is increased and followed by the Metabolic Syndrome X [insulin resistance, abdominal obesity, elevated lipids and blood pressure]. In a minor part of the population a defect, 'burned-out' cortisol secretion occurs, with decreased sex steroid and growth hormones secretions and strong, consistent, associations with the Metabolic Syndrome X.*
>
> *Psychosocial and socioeconomic handicaps with tendencies to abuse and depressive-anxious mood changes are consistently associated... [with HPA-axis dysfunction].*
>
> *We suggest that the Metabolic Syndrome X is due to a discretely elevated cortisol secretion, discoverable during reactions to perceived stress in everyday life.*
>
> Bjorntorp, Ann MY Acad Sci, November 1999

Bjorntorp did a great deal more such work, showing exactly the same things, and other researchers have fully confirmed his findings. In my view he should have got a Nobel prize, for he proved beyond doubt that exposure to various stressors causes HPA-axis dysfunction, abnormal cortisol levels and then heart disease – precisely in that order. Has anyone outside of a small, devoted band of followers heard of him? Not likely.

The final thing I need to demonstrate is that the 'HPA-axis dysfunction response to injury' hypothesis actually fits the facts, and can explain the enormous variations in heart disease seen around the world. For the sake of brevity from now on I shall call this hypothesis, the 'stress hypothesis', as the full, accurate definition is a bit of a mouthful.

CHAPTER 10

THE STRESS HYPOTHESIS – DOES IT FIT THE FACTS?

The first task here is to see if the stress hypothesis can explain the huge variations seen in heart disease between different populations – for instance, the twenty-fold difference between Australian aboriginals and the Japanese. In addition, can the stress hypothesis explain why heart disease has waxed and waned so dramatically within populations?

For example, heart disease peaked in the USA more than fifty years ago and has been falling ever since. It is now less than one-third of the level in the 1950s. Following a very similar pattern, heart disease peaked in the UK about thirty years ago, and has been falling steadily ever since. In fact, during the latter half of the 20th century, heart disease has been going down and down in most western countries. In contrast, during the same time period, heart-disease rates have been climbing ever higher in eastern Europe.

In 1968 heart-disease rates in Czechoslovakia and France were the same. Forty years later, the Czechs – and probably the Slovaks too – had 15 times the rate in France. Today, the Ukraine has a rate of heart disease that compares unfavourably with the USA at its very worst; it is about five times the current rate in the UK, and very nearly twenty times the rate in France. But can the entire population of a country be stressed? Have the levels of stress changed dramatically over time?

Can these changes, in turn, be related to the rates of heart disease? More importantly, can any of this be proved – in any way?

Some things can never be proved. I cannot go back to the USA in the 1950s and measure HPA-axis dysfunction. Nor can I go back to the UK in the 1970s to do the same thing. What I am going to do, however, is to present a hypothesis about the main 'stressor' that causes heart disease – at the level of entire populations. Then I am going to support it using both historical and present data. The hypothesis is as follows:

The most deadly long-term stressor that can affect entire populations is something that I define as 'social dislocation' – something that as a concept, needs some further explanation. The most straightforward example of social dislocation would be something like ethnic cleansing, whereby a population is forced from their homes at the point of a gun then herded elsewhere. During this process, social and family networks are severely disrupted; family members lose touch – or are killed. Many people find themselves in a different country where they may not speak the language.

Social dislocation need not be as clear-cut as ethnic cleansing, and it can even occur without a population moving at all. Australian Aboriginals, for example, have remained in Australia. However their culture, their lifestyle, their status and their communities have been completely shredded. They now subsist at the bottom of the social hierarchy, with little sense of belonging. They have not physically left their country, but their community has been torn out from under them. Destruction of community can also be seen in other Aboriginal communities, such as the Maoris in New Zealand and Native Americans in the USA and Canada.

On the other hand, social dislocation can be as straightforward as migration to another country. Of course, migration need not be that much of a stressor. A white, Christian, middle-class lecturer moving from Oxford to Harvard is likely to find that most things remain much the same for him or her. And while there may be some sense of temporary disruption, there is unlikely to be any long-term social dislocation. For migration to create a genuine sense of social dislocation, it has to be accompanied by other factors, such as moving to an 'alien' culture. This is what happens when, say, an Asian Indian emigrates to a predominantly Christian society such as the UK, USA or Australia. The resultant cultural incompatibility will make it considerably more difficult for such migrants to fit into the surrounding social mores and customs, and gain a sense of being part of a wider community. Indeed, migrants, such as Turks in Germany, or Algerians in France, or Asians in the UK, are often subjected to other major stressors such as racism, lack of job security, language difficulties etc. Their status within the host country is often very low.

The last form of social dislocation I want to look at is when an entire society, or population, is forced to undergo massive change. Most of eastern Europe, for example, has been in a state of turmoil since WWII. Poland, just to take one example, was effectively shifted a hundred miles west, through the re-drawing of its borders. Lithuania, Estonia and Latvia were forced to take in millions of Russian workers that they didn't want – and who, equally, didn't want to be in those countries.

In fact, throughout eastern Europe people were forcibly moved between, and within, communities. At the same time, religion was stomped on, churches closed, secret-police organisations set up. All of which would have had a major negative impact on social networks and support. Then, in the late 1980s, communism began to lose its grip, the Wall came down, and the entire Soviet block was plunged into even greater chaos.

That's the basic description of the main types of social dislocation. So where's the evidence that it causes heart disease?

SOCIAL DISLOCATION AND HEART DISEASE – AN INTERNATIONAL COMPARISON

Finland – highest rate of heart disease in the 1960s/early 1970s

In the 1960s and early 1970s, Finland had the highest rate of heart disease in the world. Indeed, the country became the epicentre of heart-disease research for a while.

I'd imagine that most people would think of Finland as being a fairly cohesive society, not a country that has been swamped by migrants, or one that has undergone great social upheavals. It seems a tad on the bleak and windswept side to tempt that many people as a dream destination – I've been there once and, although I am Scottish, I found it pretty bloody harsh. So what happened to Finland?

Well, after WWII, Russia decided to claim (they called it 're-claim') a large part of Finland called Karelia. This was a time when what Russia wanted, Russia got. The result was that, in 1948, a large part of Finland was handed over to Russia, and the Finns living in this area were forced to relocate back into Finland. Some 400,000 of them. This has been described as the greatest proportional 'forced' relocation of any people in the history of Europe.

How many people outside of Finland know about this? About two, and I'm one of them. But the information is all there in black and white. Just type 'Finland', 'Karelia' and '1948' into a search engine of your choice and bingo! – go read.

To the best of my knowledge no one, at any time, has ever suggested that this massive forced relocation had anything whatsoever to do with the subsequent precipitous rise in heart disease. No one in Finland, no one in the WHO, no one anywhere. This despite the fact that the North Karelia region of Finland – where the majority of those forced out of Russia ended up – had the highest rate of heart disease of any region in Finland.

This, to me, is like finding a whole bunch of people with radiation sickness in and around Hiroshima and failing to recognise that possibly, just possibly, it might have had something to do with the huge atomic bomb that got dropped on it. Hello guys, cause and effect?

The Finns, by the way, have convinced themselves that their super-high rate of heart disease was mainly due to a bad diet, and that they got rid of heart disease by educating their population on healthy eating, also taking exercise, stopping smoking and suchlike. I am sure that this has had some effect, but they were doing exactly the same things in Sweden, and the rate of heart disease went up there.

Additionally, the main focus of the massive Finnish health intervention trial was done in North Karelia as part of the 'North Karelia Project'. Yet heart-disease rates fell much more rapidly in the neighbouring region of Kuipio, which was being used as the 'control' region, i.e. no health interventions – at all. Of course, this finding has been totally swept under the carpet, but it never fails to amuse me.

To my mind, it is clear why Finland had the highest rate of heart disease in the world in the 1960s and early 1970s. Fifteen or twenty years earlier they had suffered, proportionally, the greatest forced relocation in the history of Europe.

Scotland – highest rate of heart disease in the 1970s/early 1980s

There was a time in the 1970s when Scotland had the highest rate of heart disease in the world. The rate was far worse in the west of Scotland than the east. Everyone points to the predilection of Glaswegians for fried Mars bars and the like, as the reason for their very high rate of heart disease.

What no one points to is the fact that Glasgow is the only major city in Britain to have dramatically shrunk. If I may quote from a website called Glasgow Architecture:

Glasgow Council Housing – History

In 1946, a plan was published by the Clyde Valley Regional Planning Advisory Committee, which had been set up during the war.

It suggested the dispersal of 550,000 Glaswegians into New Towns at East Kilbride, Cumbernauld, Bishopton and Houston. Glasgow at that time had a population of around 1,130,000. [The population is now 675,000 – my note.]

So, the great and wise planners decided to demolish the tenements, and shift 550,000 Glaswegians elsewhere. Of course, this was done after a full consultation process with all 550,000… not.

And what delights awaited the half a million Scots who were relocated from Glasgow during the 1950s and 1960s? Well, here is a description of one of the glorious 'new towns' called Cumbernauld. This taken from *The Scotsman* (a Scottish newspaper):

> *Criticism of Cumbernauld, created in 1956 for the Glasgow 'overspill', usually comes from outsiders. Its stark architecture has few fans and it was described as one of the worst places to live in the UK.* The Idler's Book of Crap Towns *said 'town-planning students visit Cumbernauld to learn what not to do'.*
>
> *Before that, a business magazine awarded Cumbernauld the Carbuncle Award, bestowed annually on a town deemed to be a blot on the landscape. The town centre was described as 'a rabbit warren on stilts, a sprawling, angular concrete complex that is soulless, inaccessible, like something from Eastern Europe'.*

To be frank, I think they were being polite. I get depressed just driving past.

Now, I have to admit that the tenements of Glasgow were pretty awful. You can read Billy Connolly's biography to get some feel for just how physically awful they were. There was a sense of community and pride there too, though; people knew each other and looked out for each other (so I am reliably informed). There was a strong sense of 'belonging'.

However, when the tenements were cleared out the people were moved to some of the most dreary, drab, centrally planned, monstrous high-rise blocks of putrescent concrete ever seen. They still scar the landscape and skyline of Scotland. And they scarred the communities too.

I can assure you that there is nothing in the entire scope of human existence that lays a dead hand upon the soul more effectively than a high-rise flat in Scotland. They are disgustingly ugly, utilitarian and soulless, and they succeeded in obliterating any sense of community, or pride, in those who had the desperate misfortune to inhabit them.

To quote from Glasgow's official website:

In 1947, a delegation from Glasgow visited Marseilles to see the new 'tower blocks' designed by the French architect Le Corbusier, and a high-rise policy was hastily introduced to Glasgow. However, the planners failed to realise that this style was not suitable for all environments and people. Very quickly many high-rise developments deteriorated into dingy, ill-kempt dwellings with resulting problems of social exclusion and despair for the occupants.

As the high-rise flats went up, the old stone tenements came down, victims of the wreckers' ball in an ill-co-ordinated policy of slum clearance, and damaging local communities in the process. For example, the old Gorbals, captured in the evocative photographs of Oscar Marzaroli, might have been impoverished and rundown, but Marzaroli's snaps show children playing, neighbours talking on the pavement, and women 'hingin oot the windae'. For all the material poverty there was a genuine local pride and community spirit.

Contrast the Gorbals 'New Town' of the 1960s and 70s, epitomised by the Sir Basil Spence designed Queen Elizabeth flats, an eyesore for miles around until their demolition in the 1990s.

So a big 'three cheers' to the socialist planning czars who forced more than half a million people to move. (Sorry, but attempts at social engineering by the self-appointed elite make me very mad indeed.)

Anyway, during the 1950s and 1960s, more than half a million people were forcibly relocated from Glasgow to go and live in a world of soulless concrete, and made-up 'crap' towns. In the process, any sense of community sprit was stripped bare leading to 'social exclusion and despair'.

All of this was followed by a vertiginous rise in the rate of heart disease, which peaked some 15 to 20 years later – and has fallen ever since. Although it has to be said that parts of Glasgow, and the glorious new towns, remain utterly bleak and soulless, and within certain areas the life expectancy is 20 years less than the UK average. That's right – 20 years.

Roseto – no heart disease at all

Few people have heard of Roseto in Pennsylvania, but it makes an interesting footnote in the history of heart disease. This community was made up almost entirely of Italian immigrants who, in turn, came almost entirely from a Sicilian town called Roseto Valfortore.

So, emigration to a new country followed by a massive rise in heart disease? Ah, no. Emigration followed by a very low rate of heart disease. Why? By way of an answer, I can do no better than to reproduce the entire abstract from a paper called 'The Roseto effect: a 50-year comparison of mortality rates':

The Roseto Effect

OBJECTIVES: Earlier studies found striking differences in mortality from myocardial infarction between Roseto, a homogeneous Italian-American community in Pennsylvania, and other nearby towns between 1955 and 1965. These differences disappeared as Roseto became more 'Americanized' in the 1960s. The present study extended the comparison over a longer period of time to test the hypothesis that the findings from this period were not due to random fluctuations in small communities.

METHODS. We examined death certificates for Roseto and Bangor from 1935 to 1985. Age-standardized death rates and mortality ratios were computed for each decade.

RESULTS. Rosetans had a lower mortality rate from myocardial infarction over the course of the first 30 years, but it rose to the level of Bangor's following a period of erosion of traditionally cohesive family and community relationships. This mortality-rate increase involved mainly younger Rosetan men and elderly women.

> **CONCLUSIONS. The data confirmed the existence of consistent mortality differences between Roseto and Bangor during a time when there were many indicators of greater social solidarity and homogeneity in Roseto**

Which goes to show that migration is not necessarily deadly. What kills you is the break-up of the surrounding community.

USA – first country to suffer an epidemic of heart disease

Having mentioned Roseto, I think I should briefly look at the rest of the USA, which was the first country in modern times to suffer an extremely high rate of heart disease.

Although the statistics are not entirely robust, mainly due to the fact that the diagnosis of CHD did not exist until 1948, it is likely that the rate of heart disease rose rapidly during the 1920s and 1930s, peaked some time in the late 1940s and has fallen ever since. I do not think it is any coincidence that this followed a period during which the USA took in more immigrants than any other country in the history of the world. From 1905 to 1914, one million immigrants per year arrived in the USA. Then, in the 1920s, 1930s and 1940s, the rate of heart disease shot up. Since then it has gradually fallen.

This is a pattern that is exactly repeated in other countries that took in huge waves of immigrants. After WWII, Australia and New Zealand took in (proportionally) a huge number of immigrants. The rate of heart disease in both these countries rose rapidly, peaking in the 1970s, before gradually falling.

The Japanese – you see, it isn't genetics

The Japanese have a very low rate of heart disease ('It must be genetic…' Oh do shut up).

However, when the Japanese move to other countries they (usually) lose their protection against heart disease. Most people have put this increase in heart disease down to the fact that when the Japanese migrate they change their super-healthy diet of raw fish, and other such inedible stuff, to fast-food hamburgers – thus causing cholesterol levels to rise. Everyone, it seems, apart from Professor Michael Marmot – the man who runs the Whitehall Study.

Professor Marmot has made a number of studies on the Japanese. He looked at the rising cholesterol levels in Japan and made the following observation in the International Journal of Epidemiology: *'Considerable increases in total serum cholesterol levels do not offer an explanation of the recent decline in mortality from coronary heart disease in Japan.'* So much, then, for the fast-food conjecture.

In fact, Michael Marmot has long since recognised that the classic risk factors do not remotely explain heart-disease rates, in any population. He was also the first to demonstrate that among the Japanese – as with the Rosetans – retaining your culture is what protects you from heart disease. As he wrote in the *American Journal of Epidemiology*, as far back as 1976:

> To test the hypothesis that social and cultural differences may account for the CHD differences between Japan and the United States, 3,809 Japanese-Americans in California were classified according to the degree to which they retained a traditional Japanese culture. The most traditional group of Japanese-Americans had a CHD prevalence as low as that observed in Japan. The group that was most acculturated to Western culture had a three- to five-fold excess in CHD prevalence. This difference in CHD rate between most and least acculturated groups could not be accounted for by the differences in the major coronary risk factors.

I have done a bit more hunting on the Japanese, and several other interesting facts emerge. The first is that Japanese Americans have a much higher rate of type II diabetes (adult onset diabetes) than native Japanese. In fact, a study in Brazil found that Japanese migrants had a rate of type II diabetes that was ten times higher than that in Japan. Type II diabetes is a key indicator of HPA-axis dysfunction.

Importantly though, this effect is not seen in Japanese migrants who retain a Japanese lifestyle. In 1996, Dr Boji Huang of the University of

Hawaii's Honolulu Heart Program did a study on Japanese-American men living in Hawaii. He found that '*A reduced prevalence of diabetes was observed among the men who had retained a more Japanese lifestyle. These findings suggest that living a Japanese lifestyle is associated with a reduced prevalence of diabetes.*'

Marmot himself wrote that '*Japanese culture is characterized by a high degree of social support. There is evidence that this may contribute to the low rate of heart disease in Japan, and among Japanese-Americans who retain their traditional culture.*'

On the other hand, studies have shown that 'non-accultured' Japanese Americans are much more prone to develop visceral obesity, insulin resistance (diabetes), dyslipidaemia (high VLDL, low HDL) hypertension and coronary heart disease than native Japanese.

At which point it is time to move from the area of hypothesis to the area of hard data.

SOCIAL DISLOCATION AND THE PHYSICAL MARKERS OF HPA-AXIS DYSFUNCTION

While social dislocation cannot be measured, it can be demonstrated that in populations that I would consider to be 'dislocated' there are a whole series of measurable metabolic abnormalities to be found. All of which point, in big bright neon lights, straight towards HPA-axis dysfunction.

I could look at many populations, but I will restrict myself to three:

1: Australian Aboriginals
2: Asian Indian emigrants
3: Eastern Europeans

1: Australian Aboriginals

> *Rapid social and lifestyle changes have been very important in the poor health status of Aboriginals. They are also subject to severe socio-economic discrimination, underemployment, limited education, overcrowding, social depression and severely depressed housing conditions, relative inaccessibility to adequate*

and nutritious foodstuffs, and limited access to clinical services. Aboriginal people are prone to obesity, hypertension, type-2 diabetes mellitus and cardiovascular diseases.

Gracey, M. 'A pediatrician and his mothers
and infants', Turk J Pediatr, 1997

Australian Aboriginals also suffer very high rates of depression and suicide. They have a rate of type II diabetes (a sure sign of HPA-axis dysfunction) of 21 per cent. This compares with around 3 per cent in the UK. They also show clear signs of excess cortisol secretion. Look under 'Schmitt, Harrison and Spargo' for several papers in this area on the pubmed website.

Aboriginals also have high levels of abdominal/visceral obesity, high VLDL levels, low HDL levels and a very high rate of hypertension – often leading to kidney failure. The life expectancy of an Australian aboriginal is 20 years less than that of the surrounding 'European Australians'.

Of the utmost irony, with regard to Australian Aboriginals, is that the only health intervention that seems to have been put into action is the advice to reduce saturated-fat consumption. And it's true that their cholesterol levels have dropped a bit. However, in this population a high blood cholesterol – defined as being above 5.5mmol/l – is associated with by far the lowest risk of dying of heart disease. This is one reference that I will provide, as it is a bit difficult to find[11].

In fact, in those with high cholesterol levels, the risk of dying of heart disease is 0.29 compared to those with low cholesterol levels – who had a comparative risk of 1. Or, to put this another way, an Australian Aboriginal with a high cholesterol level is more than three times less likely to die of heart disease than an Australian Aboriginal with a low cholesterol level. So, keep up the dietary advice, guys, and see how many more you can kill.

Personally, I don't think that there can be any doubt that the main cause of heart disease in Australian Aboriginals is an extreme form of

11 Robyn McDermott et al, 'Increase in prevalence of obesity and diabetes and decrease in plasma cholesterol in a central Australian Aboriginal community', MJA 2000.

social dislocation. They demonstrate every single step from unhealthy stressor, through HPA-axis dysfunction to heart disease. And if you can come up with another reason as to why they have such a high rate of heart disease, then please let me know.

2: Emigrant Asian Indians
It has long been known that Asian Indian emigrants suffer very high rates of heart disease. As I mentioned earlier in the book, this is despite the fact that many of them are vegetarian and rates of smoking in this community are often very low, as are the levels of obesity (at least measured by the body mass index, or BMI).

A study entitled 'Coronary heart disease and its risk factors in first-generation immigrant Asian Indians to the United States of America', headed by Dr EA Enas, found that the immigrants had three times the rate of heart disease and eight times the rate of type II diabetes, along with a whole series of other metabolic abnormalities that can be traced straight back to HPA-axis dysfunction:

> To conclude, immigrant Asian Indian men to the US have high prevalence of CHD, NIDDM [type II diabetes], low HDL cholesterol levels and hypertriglyceridaemia [high VLDL]. All these have 'insulin resistance' as a common pathogenetic mechanism and seem to be the most important risk factors.

In fact, wherever you look, you find the same things in Emigrant Asian Indians. Diabetes, insulin resistance, visceral-fat deposition, high VLDL, low HDL, high Lp(a) et cetera, et cetera. Just to give one last quote from a UK study done by Marmot, Shah and McKeigue and published in *The Lancet* in 1991:

> In comparison with the European group, the South Asian group had a higher prevalence of diabetes (19% vs 4%), higher blood pressures, higher fasting and post-glucose serum insulin concentrations, higher plasma triglyceride, and lower HDL

*cholesterol concentrations. Mean waist-hip girth ratios and trunk
skinfolds were higher in the South Asian than in the European
group. Within each ethnic group waist-hip ratio was correlated
with glucose intolerance, insulin, blood pressure, and triglyceride.
These results confirm the existence of an insulin resistance
syndrome, prevalent in South Asian populations and associated
with a pronounced tendency to central obesity in this group.*

Some researchers have even looked at cortisol levels in Asian emigrants.
Unfortunately, most of them persist in doing one measurement at 8 a.m.
or 9 a.m. Unsurprisingly, therefore, they keep finding low levels of cortisol.
For example, a study carried out in Edinburgh and published May 2006
noted: 'Cortisol levels are lower in South Asian than in European men
resident in the UK. Despite lower cortisol levels in South Asians, the
relations between cortisol and cardiovascular risk factors remain strong.'
Bong! Wrong answer. Please go and read Bjorntorp's work in this area.

Are you convinced yet? Personally, I cannot believe that this research
has not been brought together before. To my mind, the true underlying
cause of heart disease is 'stress' and it's standing right in front of
everyone, jumping up and down, going 'Hello, look here, it's me!... Will
you please ignore LDL levels... I SAID LOOK OVER HERE! Oh forget it...'

Anyway. It is time to turn to my final population. Which is a big one.
It's eastern Europe.

3: Eastern Europe

I am not going to look at the whole of eastern Europe, you will be
pleased to know. Just a few bits. Firstly, I'll attempt to convey the scale
of the problem, which is quite frightening. This from a paper published
in the *Journal of the American Medical Association* in 1998:

*Russian life expectancy has fallen sharply in the 1990s, but the
impact of the major causes of death on that decline has not been
measured. Age-adjusted mortality in Russia rose by almost 33%
between 1990 and 1994. During that period, life expectancy for*

Russian men and women declined dramatically from 63.8 and 74.4 years to 57.7 and 71.2 years respectively... More than 75% of the decline in life expectancy was due to increased mortality rates for ages 25 to 64 years. Increases in cardiovascular mortality accounted for 41.6% of the decline in life expectancy for women and 33.4% for men.

The striking rise in Russian mortality is beyond the peacetime experience of industrialized countries, with a 5 year decline in life expectancy in 4 years time. Many factors appear to be acting simultaneously, including economic and social instability, high rates of tobacco and alcohol consumption, poor nutrition, depression, and deterioration of the health care system. Problems in data quality and reporting appear unable to account for these findings.

Male Russian life expectancy is now *20 years* less than that in most of western Europe. And this pattern can be seen across eastern Europe: Latvia, Lithuania, Poland, the Ukraine. You name an eastern European country – after the Wall came down they were all plunged into a health crisis. In truth, Poland seems to be emerging from the other side, and heart-disease rates have been falling for more than ten years. Hopefully, the other countries will soon be following suit.

One group of researchers decided to find out what was behind this unprecedented rise in heart disease. They decided to look at men living in Sweden and Lithuania. What's more, they decided to measure the differences in 'psychosocial strain'. I can do no better than to reprint the abstract, because the findings could not be more clear:

Increased psychosocial strain in Lithuanian versus Swedish men (the LiVicordia Study)

OBJECTIVE: Coronary heart disease (CHD) mortality is four times higher in 50-year-old Lithuanian men than in 50-year-old Swedish men. The difference cannot be explained by standard risk factors. The objective of this study was to

examine differences in psychosocial risk factors for CHD in the two countries.

METHODS: The LiVicordia study is a cross-sectional survey comparing 150 randomly selected 50-year-old men in each of the two cities: Vilnius, Lithuania, and Linkoping, Sweden. As part of the study, a broad range of psychosocial characteristics, known to predict CHD, were investigated.

RESULTS: In the men from Vilnius compared with those from Linkoping, we found a cluster of psychosocial risk factors for CHD; higher job strain, lower social support at work, lower emotional support, and lower social integration. Vilnius men also showed lower coping, self-esteem, and sense of coherence, higher vital exhaustion, and depression. Quality of life and perceived health were lower and expectations of ill health within 5 to 10 years were higher in Vilnius men. Correlations between measurements on traditional and psychosocial risk factors were few and weak.

CONCLUSIONS: The Vilnius men, representing the population with a four-fold higher CHD mortality, had unfavourable characteristics on a cluster of psychosocial risk factors for CHD in comparison with the Linkoping men. We suggest that this finding may provide a basis for possible new explanations of the differences in CHD mortality between Lithuania and Sweden.

The investigators then went one step further. They measured the levels of cortisol, in response to a standard stress test. Thirty minutes after the stress was applied the change in baseline cortisol level was five times greater in the Swedish men than the Lithuanian men (88.4nmol/1 vs 18.1nmol/1). In their words:

A low peak cortisol response was significantly related to high baseline cortisol, current smoking, and vital exhaustion. The findings suggest a physiological mechanism of chronic psychosocial stress, which may contribute to increased risk for cardiovascular death.

Right is that enough for you? If you don't believe that social dislocation causes heart disease by now, I'll never be able to convince you.

CHAPTER 11

OTHER FORMS OF STRESS

Before signing off, I would like to present some of the evidence pointing to the fact that stressors, other than social dislocation, cause heart disease. Also, that short-term stressors, e.g. cocaine use, trigger the final, fatal thrombosis.

What follows is a rather eclectic list of stressors. The main point I am trying to get across here is that – in the end – everything links back to the impact that stressors have on the HPA-axis. And when I say everything, I mean everything.

POSITION IN SOCIAL HIERARCHY

With psychological stress, some people have found it useful to define damaging stress as the type of stress that makes you feel trapped, that you have no control over. This has been lumped under the heading 'man in a box'. This means that the worst types of psychological stress are often found in those low down the social hierarchy. Untouchables in India, or migrants living in another country, or Australian Aboriginals, or people who do jobs that are held in contempt by others in society, e.g. traffic wardens. These are 'situations' that are reactive, and oppressive, and crushing to the spirit.

On the other hand, a CEO of a company, or a prime minister, has a lot to deal with, but each can always, if they wish, stop doing it. They have money, they have status, they can get another job at any time. People defer to them, listen to them, treat them with respect. They sit atop the pile, and those who sit atop the pile are in charge of their own destiny.

It's not just human beings who are better off if they sit at the top of the pile, either. There are many studies demonstrating that dominant monkeys are protected against heart disease, while subordinate monkeys are not. Here is a quote from just one study on macaque monkeys, 'Effects of gender and social behavior on the development of coronary artery atherosclerosis in cynomolgus macaques', published in *Atherosclerosis*:

> *Males had significantly more extensive coronary artery atherosclerosis than did females. Further, among both males and females, submissive animals (low in competitiveness) had more extensive coronary artery stenosis than did their dominant (highly competitive) counterparts.*

In the monkey world, at least, it seems that Type A monkeys do rather better than Type Bs.

There is also very clear evidence that humans who sit at the top of the pile are protected against heart disease (and many other type of disease as well). The Whitehall Study, which has been going on for years, has found that civil servants in higher-ranking jobs suffer much less heart disease, and live far longer, than those further down the pecking order. This seems to be modulated, primarily, by a lack of job control. Here is just a short section from one of the many papers on the Whitehall Study, published in the *BMJ* in 1994:

> *Low control in the work environment is associated with an increased risk of future coronary heart disease among men and women employed in government offices.*

If you care to, you can find hundreds and hundreds of papers on the topic of social hierarchy, social status and heart disease. You will always find the same thing. Those low down on the ladder, be it rats, monkeys, or humans, are at far greater risk of dying of heart disease. It seems that social inequality leads, inevitably, to health inequality.

However, the Whitehall Study reveals something else rather interesting, which is that position in social hierarchy is much more important to men than it is to women:

> *Although the Whitehall II cohort is an office-based occupational cohort there seems no reason why these results should not generalize to the population at large. Altogether, the results of this study support the existing evidence that psychological distress is a risk factor for CHD, in men,* **if not in women** *[my emphasis].*

I have not, up to this point, suggested any reason why women suffer less heart disease than men – in most populations. However, at this point I am going to explain why women get less heart disease than men – in most populations.

A pedant would say that women do not get less heart disease than men, they just tend to get heart disease about ten years later. In other words, for every man that keels over of heart disease at 50, there is a women keeling over at 60. And for every man dropping dead at 60, there is a women dropping dead at 70 – and so on. Until, of course, there is no one left to drop dead of anything.

This is not true of all populations everywhere, but it is generally true. Which suggests that there is something going on in most populations that makes heart disease develop far more slowly in women. Is this caused by a difference in their 'stress response?' I believe so.

As a wise man once said – and if he didn't, he probably should have – if you watch a riot, or protests, or fights at football matches, or wars, you don't tend to see that many women involved. Major acts of hostility and aggression – they're kind of a man thing. Don't blame us, though, I think we were made that way. And while all this aggression was a good thing to have in our primitive past, it doesn't work quite so well when your most fearsome enemy is a parking attendant, or the plastic wrapper on a child's toy. Or, in fact, many of the hugely frustrating things that make up life today.

THE GREAT CHOLESTEROL CON

Beating the living daylights out of a sabre-toothed tiger was probably enormously exciting and satisfying. But we successfully beat the living daylights out of the last sabre-toothed tiger years ago and now there are none left. PlayStation is not quite the same. Which is why we men have taken to racing cars, gambling, sky-diving, boxing, rioting at football matches and suchlike. Of course there are men who don't do such things, and women that do, but it's a pretty good generalization to say that women, in general, do not react in such hostile and aggressive ways to stressors – or life in general.

In fact, I think that there are three interconnected reasons why women are protected from heart disease:

1: They are less hostile/aggressive to start with.
2: They are better at developing social support networks.
3: They respond in a physiologically different way to stressors.

Or, to put this another way, women are made of sugar and spice and everything nice. Men are made of slugs and snails and puppy dog's tails. However, is there any evidence for a real, measurable difference? Only a few hundred thousand papers, or so. Just to give you a feel for this area.

To start with, the British Heart Foundation looked at the social support, or the lack of it, between various social classes, and between men and women (see Fig. 31). As you can see, people in lower social classes felt that they had far less social support. And in all social classes, a far higher percentage of men reported a severe lack of social support.

And social networks are important. The Stockholm Female Coronary Risk Study looked at women who had suffered heart disease with a particular emphasis on integration and depression among this group. They found that women who lacked social integration – and had two or more depressive symptoms – had four times the rate of serious heart disease recurrence (up to and including death) as women who were free of these characteristics. The actual figures were 35 per cent vs 9 per cent.

Fig. 31 Percentage of people who report severe lack of social support in the UK

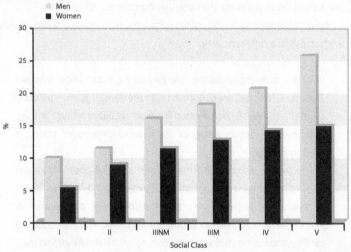

The importance of social support was strongly supported by another Swedish study (what is it about the Swedes and stress?):

> *The results of our study suggest that lack of emotional support, social isolation, and lack of interpersonal social relations are important risk factors for accelerated progression of coronary atherosclerosis in middle-aged women.*
>
> *Wang HX. 'Influence of social support on progression of coronary artery disease in women', Soc Sci Med, 2005*

And, yes, social support is also important for men:

> *In this prospective study of men, we found two dimensions of low social support – low social integration and low emotional attachment – to be predictive of coronary morbidity, independently of other risk factors.*
>
> *Rosengren A, 'Coronary disease in relation to social support and social class in Swedish men. A 15 year follow-up in the study of men born in 1933', Eur Heart J, 2004*

In short, social support is very important at protecting against heart disease. In general, women have much better social networks than men. But I don't suppose that you needed me to tell you this.

Apart from having better social networks, women also seem to deal with stress in a different way.

Why are men more susceptible to heart disease than women? Traditional risk factors cannot explain the gender gap in coronary heart disease (CHD) or the rapid increase in CHD mortality among middle-aged men in many of the newly independent states of Eastern Europe.

However, Eastern European men score higher on stress-related psychosocial factors than men living in the West. Comparisons between the sexes also reveal differences in psychosocial and behavioral coronary risk factors favoring women, indicating that women's coping with stressful events may be more cardioprotective.

Weidner G, 'The gender gap in heart disease: lessons from Eastern Europe', Am J Public Health, 2003

Few studies have focused on risk factors in women's lives concerning psychosocial factors and coronary heart disease (CHD)… Significant differences appeared concerning five areas: work content, workload and control, physical stress reactions, emotional stress reactions and burnout. All showed that the relative sensitivity was larger for women than for men.

Predictive psychosocial risk factors for women with respect to CHD were physical stress reactions, emotional stress reactions, burnout, family relationships and daily hassles/satisfactions, and they were on approximately the same level as biomedical risk factors.

Women appear to be more sensitive than men with respect to psychosocial risk factors for CHD, and the predictive ability of psychosocial risk factors shows great importance. Actions against unhealthy psychosocial conditions are recommended. Both presumptive CHD patients and others might benefit from preventive actions, and since women are more sensitive they will probably gain more than men.

Hallman T, 'Psychosocial risk factors for coronary heart disease, their importance compared with other risk factors and gender differences in sensitivity', J Cardiovasc Risk, 2001

However, it is not just better social networks and superior coping mechanisms that make the difference. It is clear that men, when exposed to the same type of psychological stressor, have a much more violent HPA-axis reaction.

A study in Germany published in the *Journal of Clinical Endocrinology and Metabolism* showed that, when stressed, men produce nearly twice as much ACTH as women. (ACTH is the precursor hormone that triggers the release of cortisol (see Fig. 32)).

Fig. 32 Comparison of ACTH produced by men and women in stressful situations

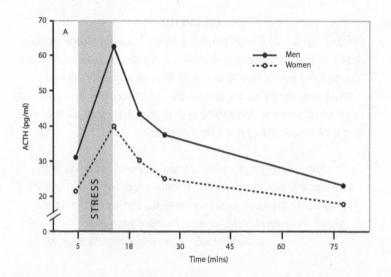

You see, us poor men are at the mercy of our hormones too. The difference is that our hormones kill us – if we haven't killed someone else first. 'Get your finger off that button, Mr President.'

For whatever reason, and I can think of many, men respond more dramatically to stressors. We fire up our stress hormones far more powerfully and we find it harder to get things back under control again. By way of illustrating this, here's a quote from a study called 'Gender differences in hypothalamic-pituitary-adrenal (HPA) axis reactivity':

> *Following the psychological stressor, adrenocorticotropin (ACTH)*
> *and cortisol responses were significantly greater in male subjects*
> *compared to female subjects.*

In summary, women are better at recognising that they are stressed and have better coping mechanisms. Their HPA-axes are not provoked into such a violent reactions by stress, and if they are, they have a better network of social support then men to cope with think. Maybe it's time for us guys to get in touch with our feminine side?

COCAINE USE

Cocaine has a major impact on the heart. It causes sudden cardiac death, angina and myocardial infarction. While this is an undisputed finding, most authorities do not know how, or why, this happens.

What they ought to do is type the words 'cocaine and HPA-axis dysfunction' into a search engine of their choice. They would then find all the information they need. For example:

> *Scientists have been aware of the existence of a complex*
> *relationship between stress and the subsequent activation of the*
> *hypothalamic-pituitary-adrenal (HPA) axis and the endocrine and*
> *neurobehavioral effects of cocaine for many years now.*
>
> Goeders NE, Psychoneuroendocrinology, 2002

The fact is that cocaine is one of the most powerful stimulants of the HPA-axis known to man. Cocaine use burns out the HPA-axis, it causes depression, it creates blood clotting abnormalities. Taking it is almost the perfect way to kill yourself from heart disease, and it can occur very quickly. To quote from www.ScienceDaily.com:

> During the first hour after using cocaine, the user's risk of heart attack increases nearly 24 times, according to the first large study of the long-suspected relationship between cocaine and heart disease. The research is reported in today's Circulation: Journal of the American Heart Association.

And some people try to tell me that stress doesn't cause heart disease, or trigger fatal heart attacks.

FOOTBALL – A MATTER OF LIFE AND DEATH

Rather surprisingly, some researchers decided to look at the impact of football on the rates of death from heart disease. In 2003, a study was published in the *Journal of Epidemiology and Public Health* called 'A matter of life and death: population mortality and football results'. And what did they find?

> On days when the local professional football team lost at home, mortality attributable to acute myocardial infarction and stroke increased significantly in men. No increase was observed in women.

However, when France won the World Cup in 1998, there was a considerably lower mortality from heart attacks the next day – as written up in a paper called 'Lower myocardial infarction mortality in French men the day France won the 1998 World Cup of football', and published in *Heart*.

By the way, this is not fringe research. A study was published in the *BMJ* in 2002 called 'Admissions for myocardial infarction and World Cup football: database survey', which revealed that:

Risk of admission for acute myocardial infarction increased by 25% on 30 June 1998 [the day England lost to Argentina in a penalty shoot-out] and the following two days. No excess admissions occurred for other diagnoses or on the days of the other England matches.

To misquote Bill Shankly: 'Football isn't just a matter of life and death... It is life and death.'

Golly, you mean that the stress of watching your football team lose can kill you? Well, so can getting up on a Monday morning...

MONDAY MORNINGS – DON'T GET OUT OF BED

As published in the *European Journal of Cardiology* in 2003:

> *The incidence of sudden cardiac death is markedly increased on Monday, more pronounced in non-hospitalised patients. Our results may point to the relevance of naturally occurring rhythmic fluctuations in human physiology, and socially determined rhythms in human behaviour as underlying mechanism.*

So the number four doesn't wipe out us westerners, but Mondays do. In Japan, though – if you are a woman – Saturdays are deadly. I wonder why? Isn't marriage a wonderful thing...

Leaving Monday mornings behind for a moment, wherever you look you will find the same things. Stressful events, be they physical or psychological, greatly increase the risk of dying of heart disease. For example, a study published in the *British Heart Journal* in 1975 found the following:

> *The deaths of 100 men due to coronary artery disease which occurred so suddenly and unexpectedly as to merit a coroner's necropsy have been studied, with special reference to the exact circumstances of their occurrence. The most significant relationship of sudden death was with acute psychological stress.*

Here follows a short list of some of the other things that have been found to increase the risk:

- Shovelling snow after a blizzard
- Being a fighter-jet pilot
- Earthquakes
- Squash
- Exposure to congestedtraffic (three-fold increased risk of MI in the next 24 hours)
- Rapid temperature change
- Cold weather
- Episode of severe anger (risk increased 15-fold in the following hour)

Wherever you look, you will find that hundreds, even thousands, of studies have been done. They all show exactly the same thing. Stress causes heart disease. It can be long term, it can be short term, it can be physical or psychological. It doesn't matter, the HPA-axis converts all types of stress into the same deadly mix.

Ironically, of course, this was all recognised hundreds of years ago. In 1628, William Harvey, the man who first worked out how the cardiovascular system worked, described a man with heart disease as: 'Overcome with anger and indignation and unable to communicate it to anyone.' In 1793 John Hunter, the most famous physician of his time, believed that angina was related to 'agitation of the mind'. He died suddenly in a stormy board meeting the very same year. It is thought that he died of a heart attack. At the start of the 20th century, William Osler, another eminent physician, described the typical victim of heart disease as:

> A well set man from forty-five to fifty five years of age, with military bearing and iron grey or florid complexion. Robust and vigorous of mind and body whose engine is always at full ahead.

Oh yes, heart disease has been with humanity for many years. It is not new. In fact, it was perfectly described by the 18th-century London physician William Heberden. In 1772, he first outlined the condition that he called angina pectori:

Heberden's description of angina

But there is a disorder of the breast marked with strong and peculiar symptoms, considerable for the kind of danger belonging to it, and not extremely rare, which deserves to be mentioned at more length. The seat of it and the sense of strangling and anxiety with which it is attended, may make it not improperly be called angina pectoris.

Those who are afflicted with it are seized while they are walking (more especially if it be uphill, and soon after eating) with a painful and most disagreeable sensation of the breast, which seems as if it would extinguish life if it were to increase or to continue. But the moment they stand still, all this uneasiness vanishes.

In all other respects the patients are, at the beginning of this disorder, perfectly well, and in particular have no shortness of breath, from which it is totally different. The pain is sometimes situated in the upper part, sometimes in the middle, sometimes in the bottom of the os sterni (breast bone), and often more inclined to the left than the right side. It likewise very frequently extends from the breast to the middle of the left arm. The pulse is, at least sometimes, not disturbed by this pain, as I have had opportunities of observing by feeling the pulse during the paroxysm. Males are more liable to this disorder, especially such as have passed their fiftieth year.

After it has continued a year of more, it will not cease so instantaneously upon standing still: and will come on not only when the person is walking, but when they are lying down, especially if they lie on the left side and oblige them to rise out of their beds. In some inveterate cases it has been

---

brought on by the motion of a horse, or a carriage, and even by swallowing, coughing, going to stool or speaking, or any disturbance of the mind

Such is the most usual appearance of this disease; but some varieties may be met with. Some have been seized while they were standing still, or sitting, also upon first waking out of sleep; and the pain sometimes reaches to the right arm, as well as to the left and even down to the hands, but this is uncommon; in a very few instances the arm has at the same time been numbed and swelled. In one or two persons the pain has lasted some hours or even days; but this has happened when the complaint has been of long standing, or thoroughly rooted in the constitution; once only the very first attack continued the whole night.

I have seen nearly a hundred people under this disorder, of which number there have been three women and one boy twelve years old. All the rest were men near or past the fiftieth year of their age.

The termination of angina pectoris is remarkable. For if no accident interferes, but the disease goes on to its height, the patients all suddenly fall down, and perish almost immediately.

And perishing almost immediately is what I am trying to help you avoid.

POSTSCRIPT

By now, I hope you know what causes heart disease, and what you may be able to do to prevent it. Some things that I have outlined are the same things that the medical mainstream has been saying for years. Do not smoke cigarettes. If you do not smoke cigarettes you will live longer, and more happily, and be considerably better off. Cigarettes are, quite frankly, pointless and deadly.

Also, take exercise. Take the type of exercise that you enjoy, join a club, go walking, do something – anything – to avoid sitting doing nothing. Human beings need some exercise; if they don't get it, they degenerate. They also become depressed, anxious and unhappy.

If you don't drink alcohol, start. If you do drink, drink regularly – don't binge drink – and make sure you enjoy what you drink. Drink with friends, drink sociably; don't drink to get drunk.

If you hate your job, try and find another one. If you have a bully for a boss, take them to an industrial tribunal and sue their ass. Don't let anyone push you about. Don't be a victim. Don't feel trapped. Assert yourself and ensure that people give you the respect that you – indeed, all of us – deserve.

Make a new friend. Join a club. Find an area of life that you enjoy and can enjoy in the company of other people. Praise other people, and try to compliment people more often. As ye sow, so shall ye reap. Look forward to something enjoyable every day, every month and every year.

Does this sound like a list of homilies? A tea towel for the soul? I hope not, or if it does, I hope it does not put you off doing what you need to do. What you always knew you should do, in fact.

Everyone has always known that stress kills. The medical profession, which has a horrible aversion to accepting that there is any connection between the mind and the body, has tried to crush this 'knowledge' using western scientific methodology as its weapon of choice. 'We can't measure stress, so it doesn't exist.'

Ironically, it is western science that proves the connection – if you choose to accept the evidence of your own eyes. The Catholic Church wouldn't look through Galileo's telescope – a fact that 'scientists' regularly use to castigate religion. Well, guys, the second half of this book has been a telescope focused on stress. All I ask you to do is look through it.

GLOSSARY

Acromegaly: a chronic disease, characterised by enlargement of the bones of the head, hands and feet and the swelling of soft tissue. This condition is caused by excessive secretion of growth hormone by the pituitary gland.

Adipose: of, relating to or containing fat.

Aneurysm: a sac formed by the extreme dilation of the wall of a blood vessel.

Angioplasty: a surgical technique for restoring normal blood flow through a blocked artery, either by inserting and inflating a balloon into the affected section or by using a laser beam.

Arrhythmia: any variation in the normal rhythm of the heartbeat.

Atheroma: a fatty deposit on or within the inner lining of an artery, which can often obstruct blood flow.

Atherosclerosis: a degenerative disease of the arteries, caused by build-up of fatty deposits on the inner lining of arterial walls.

CABG: coronary artery bypass graft.

Cerebral haemorrhage: a form of stroke caused by bleeding in the brain due to a burst artery.

CHD: coronary heart disease.

Chyle: a milky fluid consisting of lymph and emulsified fat globules. It is formed in the small intestine during digestion.

Chylomicron: a large lipoprotein that enables fatty substances to be transported in the blood and chyle.

Cis bond: part of a molecular structure featuring a double bond with hydrogen atoms on the same side.

Cohort: a group of people with a statistic in common.

Cyanosis: a bluish-purple discolouration of skin and mucous membranes, usually caused by a deficiency of oxygen in the blood.

Endocrine glands: glands that secrete hormones directly into the bloodstream. These include the pituitary, adrenal, thyroid, testes and ovaries.

Endothelium: a tissue, comprising a single layer of cells, that lines the blood and lymph vessels, the heart and other cavities.

Epidemiology: the branch of medicine concerned with the study of epidemic diseases.

Ester: any one of a class of compounds produced by reaction between acids and alcohols, with the elimination of water.

Externa: connective tissue that surrounds a blood vessel and holds it together.

Familial hypercholesterolaemia (FH): a hereditary condition of having high levels of cholesterol in the blood.

Glia: a delicate web of connective tissue surrounding and supporting nerve cells.

HDL: high density lipoprotein.

Heterozygous FH: a form of FH in which a person inherits the FH gene from one parent.

Homozygous FH: a form of FH in which a person inherits the FH gene from both parents.

HRT: hormone replacement therapy.

Hyperlipidaemia: raised cholesterol levels in the blood.

Hypertension: raised blood pressure levels

Hyponatremia: an abnormally low concentration of sodium in the blood.

Hypothalamus: a control centre at the base of the brain that is triggered by states such as hunger, thirst and fear.

IDL: intermediate density lipoprotein.

Infarction: the formation of an infarct (a localised area of dead tissue that is caused by restriction of blood flow to that area).

LCAT: lecithin cholesterol acyltransferase, an enzyme.

LDL: low density lipoprotein.

Lipid: any one of a large group of organic compounds that are esters of fatty acids.

Lipoprotein: a protein-based capsule that enables substances such as cholesterol and fats to travel within the body.

Macrophage: any large phagocytic cell in the blood, lymph and connective tissue of vertebrates.

Media: the middle layer of the wall of a blood or lymph vessel.

MI: Myocardial Infarction – a localised necrosis resulting from obstruction to the blood supply.

Necrosis: the death of body cells – usually in a localised area – often due to interruption of blood supply.

Ophthalmology: the branch of medicine relating to the eye and its diseases.

Phagocyte: an amoeboid cell or protozoan that engulfs particles such as food substances of invading microorganisms.

Phenotype: the physical constitution of an organism as determined by the interaction of its genetic constitution and the environment.

Pituitary gland: the major endocrine gland, attached to the base of the brain by a stalk. It comprises two lobes, which secrete hormones that affect development of the sex glands, skeletal growth and the functioning of the other endocrine glands.

Placebo: an inactive substance or form of therapy given to a patient, usually to compare its effects with those of a real treatment or drug.

Plaque: a thickened area in the artery walls, formed by the build-up of fatty substances.

Pleitropism: the condition of a gene of affecting more than one characteristic of the phenotype.

Smith-Lemli-Opitz Syndrome (SLOS): a medical condition characterised by extremely low cholesterol levels.

Synapse: the point at which a nerve impulse transfers from the

terminal portion of an axon – a long extension of a nerve cell that conducts nerve impulses from the cell body – to an adjacent neuron.
Thrombosis: the formation of blood clots within a blood vessel or the heart, often resulting in restricted blood flow.
Trans bond: part of a molecular structure in which a hydrogen atom sits either side of a double carbon bond.